# RADIOGRAPHY OF CHILDREN

## A GUIDE TO GOOD PRACTICE

**Judith Hardwick** DCR DMS CertPsych

*Association of Paediatric Radiographers;*
*Paediatric Radiographer; formerly Superintendent Radiographer,*
*Great Ormond Street Hospital for Children, London, UK*

**Catherine Gyll** DCR FETC

*Paediatric Radiographer; formerly of Westminster Children's Hospital,*
*London & Royal Alexandra Hospital for Sick Children, Brighton, UK*

D1338361

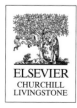

ELSEVIER
CHURCHILL
LIVINGSTONE

Edinburgh   London   New York   Oxford   Philadelphia   St Louis   Sydney   Toronto 2004

**ELSEVIER**
CHURCHILL
LIVINGSTONE

© 2004, Elsevier Limited. All rights reserved.

The right of Judith Hardwick and Catherine Gyll to be identified as authors of this work has been asserted by them in accordance with the Copyright, Designs and Patents Act 1988.

First published 2004

ISBN 0 443 07257 4

**British Library Cataloguing in Publication Data**
A catalogue record for this book is available from the British Library

**Library of Congress Cataloging in Publication Data**
A catalog record for this book is available from the Library of Congress

**Notice**
Medical knowledge is constantly changing. Standard safety precautions must be followed, but as new research and clinical experience broaden our knowledge, changes in treatment and drug therapy may become necessary or appropriate. Readers are advised to check the most current product information provided by the manufacturer of each drug to be administered to verify the recommended dose, the method and duration of administration, and contraindications. It is the responsibility of the practitioner, relying on experience and knowledge of the patient, to determine dosages and the best treatment for each individual patient. Neither the Publisher nor the authors assume any liability for any injury and/or damage to persons or property arising from this publication.

*The Publisher*

The
Publisher's
policy is to use
**paper manufactured
from sustainable forests**

Printed in China

# RADIOGRAPHY OF CHILDREN

*Digital imaging by:*

Leicester Microfilm Bureau
Brookland House
Brookland Road
Leicester. LE2 6AB


*For Elsevier*

*Associate Editor:* Dinah Thom
*Project Development Manager:* Mairi McCubbin
*Project Manager:* Morven Dean
*Designer:* Judith Wright

# Contents

# Preface

A newly qualified radiographer confronted for the first time with an uncooperative, possibly terrified, 2-year-old child from Accident and Emergency will find it a daunting experience. This patient does not fit in with anything learned about how to x-ray adult patients. Similarly, production of a high-quality chest x-ray of a tiny pre-term infant on mechanical ventilation is a highly skilled task, not always routinely achievable.

Examples of good practice in general paediatric radiography are described. We do not claim our methods to be the only way; we simply know, from long experience, that they work.

Sections on radiation protection, immobilization and child psychology are included. The final chapter reviews children's rights and important legal aspects such as restraint and consent.

We have not included fluoroscopy, computed tomography, magnetic resonance imaging or ultrasound. These imaging modalities are covered in many other publications.

The authors hope this book will be useful to students in their training, and to qualified radiographers working in general hospitals.

Judith Hardwick
Catherine Gyll

Brighton, UK, 2004

# 1 The paediatric patient

## The psychological aspects of care

A visit to a radiology department can be a nightmare for a child.

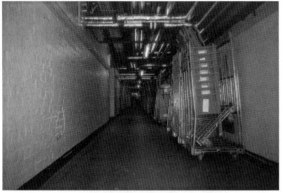

**Figure A** Where are we going to in this dark tunnel?

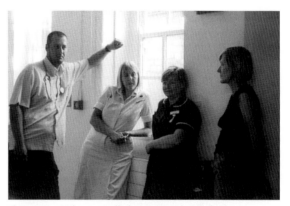

**Figure B** Who are all these people and what are they waiting for?

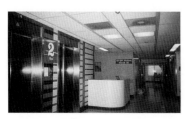

**Figure C** What's behind that high desk?

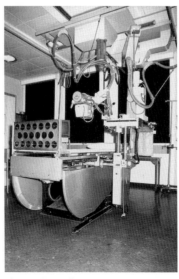

**Figure D** What a strange room.

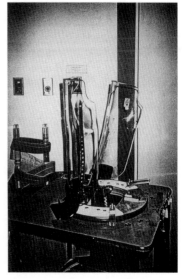

**Figure E** What is that for?

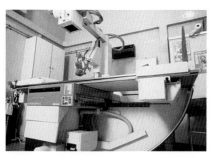

**Figure F** I'm told to climb onto the bed.

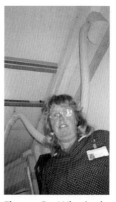

**Figure G** Why is she leaning over me?

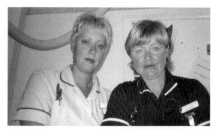

**Figure H** There are two of them now.

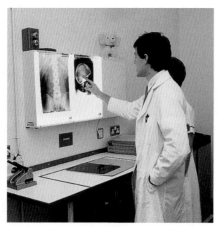

**Figure I** What are they looking at on that strange light?

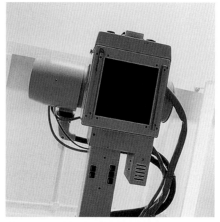

**Figure J** Why is this thing coming down on me?

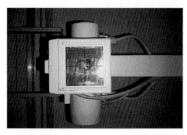

**Figure K** It's getting closer!

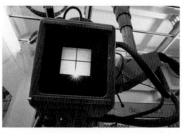

**Figure L** It's going to squash me!!!

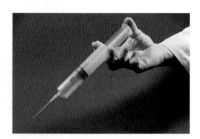

**Figure M** Is that needle going to be stuck in me?

Surely training in child psychology and its use in
immobilization techniques are preferable to this?

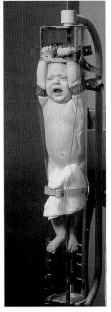

**Figure N**

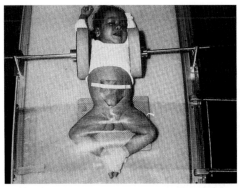

**Figure O** (Reproduced with permission from
*Die Röntgen-ulversuching in Kindersalver* by
K-D Ebel and E Willich, Abb 8 (p.12).
Copyright © Springer-Verlag, 1978.)

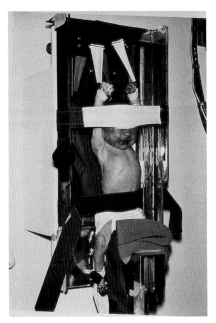

**Figure P**

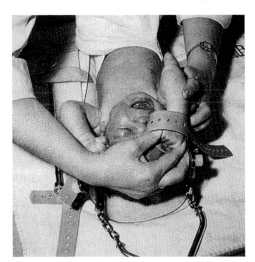

**Figure Q** (Reproduced with permission from
*Die Röntgen-ulversuching in Kindersalver* by
K-D Ebel and E Willich, Abb 142 (p.92).
Copyright © Springer-Verlag, 1978.)

**Developmental psychology**

'Experience of fear is harmful when anxiety aroused is more than a child can cope with and he is overwhelmed by it.' (Woolf, 1981)

■ Childhood experiences influence feelings that persist well into adult life, such as fear of white coats, injections, hospital smells.

■ A positive experience, making a visit as pleasant for the child as possible, will also make the examination far easier.

■ To facilitate this a radiographer must:
   ● recognize and understand the sequential stages of child development
   ● create a child-friendly environment
   ● establish a good rapport with the child and family
   ● be able to communicate and interact with children and families
   ● acknowledge that involving families in the child's examination improves patient care. Family-centred care is best practice.

**Stress factors that affect a child's psychological well-being**

Children may not have the cognitive skills to understand the experience of radiographic investigations, nor the coping skills to manage their feelings. A visit to an x-ray department almost always results in some form of anxiety. This could be caused by:
● separation from the parent or close carer, even if short-term
● strangers and new faces, such as the radiographer's
● strange environments and new experiences
● fear of needles, pain and body mutilation
● loss of independence, control (both physical and emotional) and self-esteem and limited coping strategies
● invasion of privacy and insensitivity of staff
● concerns about parental anxiety, examination viewed as punishment
   'Children's perceptions of and responses to hospital care are shaped by their age, developmental stage, and previous experience. The care that they receive in hospital profoundly affects their ability to cope with this challenging experience.' (From *Caring for Children and Families*, Association for the Care of Children's Health, 1992)
   It is possible to plan and deliver services that support the child and minimize the negative potential of an experience in the radiology department.

What is needed from a child in order to achieve a successful x-ray examination?

**The child and the radiographer**

The child should:
● co-operate when being positioned
● keep still when positioned
● follow instructions about breathing.

Reasonable adult patients comply. They accept that the examination is for their own benefit. A child does not always understand this. Even when told, children may not believe or may not comprehend, therefore they may not do what is required. How can a radiographer ensure that they do?

The child's co-operation depends on:

- age
- emotional state at the time of the examination
- degree of dependence on the parents
- secure/insecure family background and degree of socialization
- previous experiences in hospitals
- motivation to behave well
- confidence in the radiographer.

Misconceptions about a child's behaviour are not uncommon, such as 'spoilt brat' if uncooperative, 'acting like a baby' if wanting a parent, 'cry baby' if the child becomes upset; children behave better without their parents and so are easier to x-ray. These misconceptions can impede a successful examination.

**What does the child patient need from the radiographer?**

A child waiting for an x-ray examination may be:

- happily occupied playing and quite unconcerned
- tired and fractious from waiting for a long time
- scared stiff but afraid to admit it
- too ill or injured to think about anything.

In all cases, in order to gain the confidence to cope with this new situation, the child needs: reassurance, explanation, consideration.

**Explanation**

- Explain what will happen in words at the level of the child's understanding:

- What the radiographer is going to do.

- What the x-ray equipment will do: light, noise, movement.

- What a cassette is.

- Exactly what the patient is required to do, including position for area to be x-rayed.

- The child should put his/her arm in a position when shown what to do.

**Consideration**

- Awareness of the psychological and physical needs of the child at all stages of development.

- Gentle handling, especially of small babies.

- Physical comfort. This includes neonates, who do feel pain and respond positively to considerations of their comfort.

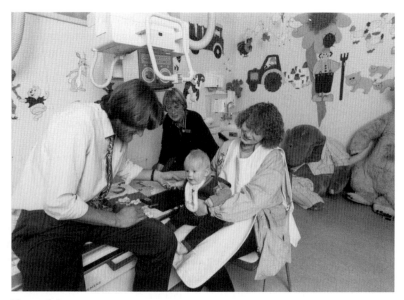

Figure 1.1

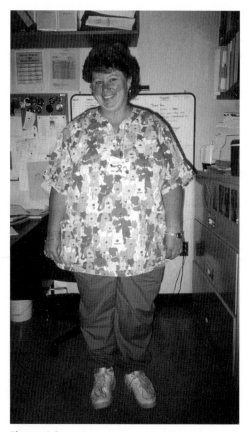

Figure 1.2

- Avoidance of distress, disturbance and pain. A sleeping baby should never be woken for an x-ray examination.

- Respect for dignity, privacy and culture.

- Respect for the child's own self-image: the child must never be humiliated, for instance by being laughed at.

- Empathy for the child's emotional state; there may be precarious control.

- Being sensitive to a child's fear or pain and not ignoring it.

- Radiographers should alter their words and actions to fit the reactions of the child.

### Reassurance

- It is not enough to say that there is nothing to fear.

- The child may need a parent: assumptions should not be made that a child is old enough to cope alone.

- Honesty: the child should not be told that 'It won't hurt' just because x-rays do not. Positioning might hurt.

- Must appear as a friendly and unthreatening radiographer: first impressions are vital (Fig. 1.1).

- There could be an alternative to a white uniform (Fig. 1.2). If this is not possible, aprons can be worn over the uniform.

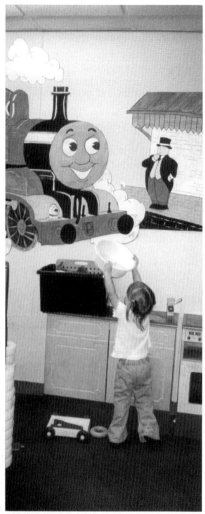

Figure 1.3a

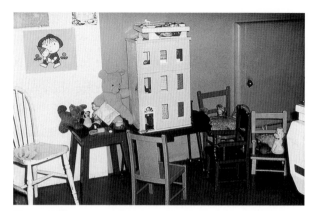

Figure 1.3b

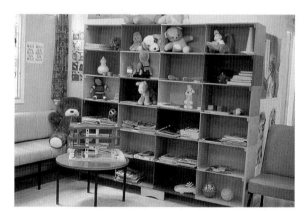

Figure 1.3c

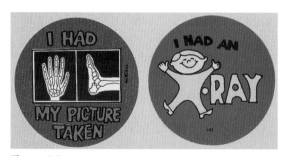

Figure 1.4

***A child-friendly environment***

- A waiting area that is bright and cheerful (Fig. 1.3a), with chairs of different sizes (Fig. 1.3b, c) and lots of appropriate things to do.

- Inducements so that the child is motivated to comply with the radiographer's instructions, such as brightly coloured stickers (Fig. 1.4) and 'Well Done' certificates or other appropriate rewards.

- An x-ray room that is not threatening. Figure 1.5a shows a typical x-ray room, which might appear very frightening to an apprehensive child. Figure 1.5b shows the same room but it is now much more patient friendly.

- With a little imagination the equipment can be disguised completely at almost no cost (Fig. 1.5c, d).

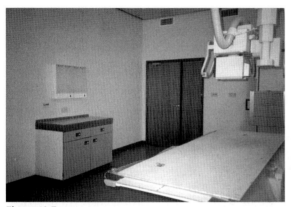

**Figure 1.5a**

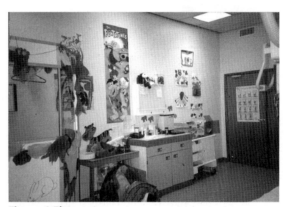

**Figure 1.5b**

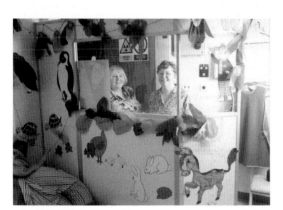

**Figure 1.5c**

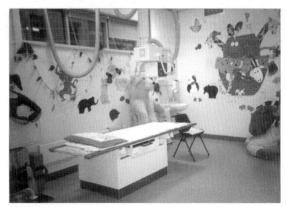

**Figure 1.5d**

**Patient care: fulfilling a child's needs**

It is impossible for radiographers to fulfil the needs of children if they do not know what these are. Friendliness, kindness and patience are not enough.

The radiographer must understand:

- how the child feels
- what causes that feeling
- what is likely to reduce/increase anxiety
- that a child may often deny feelings or not be able to put them into words.

Radiographers need to know how a child's ideas of the world, their behaviour, reactions, thoughts and feelings vary at different developmental stages throughout childhood.

When trained in **child development**, radiographers can identify or anticipate a problem; they must then be able to **communicate** with the child and family, in order to deal with it. Understanding, language, concepts, perception and attention span all vary according to age. Radiographers must be able to interpret the child's communication:

- facial expression
- body language
- spoken language (limitation of vocabulary; emotional inhibition).

They must know:

- what will reassure at different ages
- what will not even though it seems that it should, for instance picking up and cuddling a crying toddler in mother's absence.

**Child development**

Children not only grow they also develop. 'Growth is increase in size, development is change in form. This is seen throughout nature, e.g. a caterpillar develops into a chrysalis, which develops into a butterfly. At each stage a different entity, a different being, as a result of such development.' (Hadfield 1978)

- Development proceeds in stages, each following in specific order, at variable ages.

- It is the same for all races, regardless of differences in child rearing.

- Each phase is fully developed before going on to the next stage. If not, it persists into the next stage causing conflict/confusion, for instance lack of security leads to dependence on the mother at an age when the child should be independent.

'The child not only grows from infancy, through adolescence to adulthood, he also develops. If we only grew we should all be big fat babies. Maturation is development of innate patterns of behaviour in ordered sequence.' (Hadfield 1978)

Milestones of physical maturation in the first two years of life have been included for reasons of safety and radiographic positioning (ages are approximate):

- 4–6 months: can roll over, off the x-ray table
- 10 months: can crawl
- 1 year: can stand up
- 15 months: can walk
- 15–18 months: development of 'righting' mechanism, i.e. children know that they should be upright. So a child of this age, laid on the x-ray table, will automatically try to sit up, and become upset if he or she cannot.

As children cannot walk before they stand, so they cannot understand concepts or learn skills before the mind is ready to do so.

## Guide to developmental stages

### Infant (birth to 12 months)

*Behaviour*

- 0–3 months: 'startle' reflex; loud noises/sudden removal of support: baby cries
- unwrapping/leaving naked on the x-ray table causes distress
- special attachment to mother (or substitute); note how the child holds onto the mother in Fig. 1.6
- start of differentiation: self/non-self.

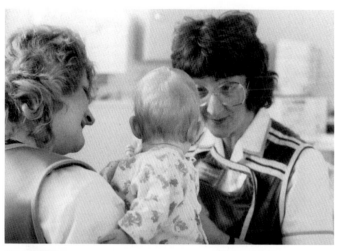

Figure 1.6

### Tips for radiographers

- 3 months: attention caught by sound, for instance music
- Up to 3 months old, babies can be wrapped in a blanket to aid immobilization. Later, wrapping up causes **upset** and **distress**.
- Position the baby so that there is always eye contact with the mother when holding.
- Think of the mother and baby as a unit whenever possible.
- Encourage the parents to help with positioning (Fig. 1.7).

### Anxiety and fears

- 6–12 months: start of memory; the child can anticipate, which may lead to anxiety. There is a common misconception that the child will forget immediately after the unpleasant experience stops
- fear of strangers/separation anxiety: normal stage 6–18 months
- loud noises in the first few months
- picking up a child of this age, to be friendly, will have an adverse reaction: it will make the child cry.

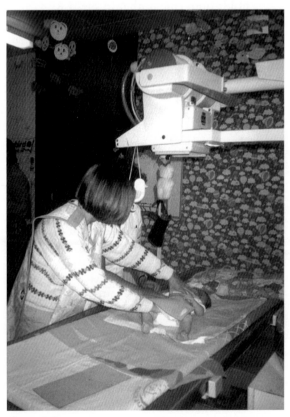

**Figure 1.7**

*Toys and distractions*
- dummy/pacifier: sucking comforts a crying baby
- games of suspense, such as 'peep-bo' with toys
- soft, squeezable, safe, washable toys
- mobiles/projected pictures on walls
- lots of colour, preferably primary (red, yellow and blue)
- music boxes/tape player.

*Preparation for examination*
- Give a full explanation to the parents in language that they will understand.
- Allow time for the parents to ask questions.
- Encourage the parents to stay with their baby but be sensitive to those who cannot stay, for whatever reason.

## Toddler (1–3 years)
*Behaviour*
- At this age, separation from the parents causes a long-lasting reaction.
- They have no sense of time, only 'now'; the child is unable to think ahead.
- Routines/rituals are important: the child gains a sense of control and learns to trust his or her environment.
- They understand words before using them.
- Thwarted desire leads to frustration/tantrums.
- They are possessive/impulsive/have no fear.
- Energetic and curious with a short attention span.

*Tips for radiographers*
- Be prepared to let toddlers do things themselves.
- Suggest that the child brings a familiar object, such as a toy from home.
- Build trust by making sure that there is something for the toddler to play with.
- Set limits/boundaries to behaviour (for safety).
- Give space to expend energy when possible in the waiting room.
- Let the child watch others being x-rayed.
- Give lots of personal attention.

*NOTE* Parental behaviour can vary from overprotective to handing over the child completely.

*Anxiety and fears*
- causality (white coat = injection)
- fear changes with what a child is able to think about
- animals/the dark (at 2+ years)
- being restrained/thwarted
- fear of noises/strange objects decreases; fear of darkness, solitude increases (at 3 years).

*Toys and distractions*
- action toys: foam blocks/safe things to climb
- simple one-to-one games such as 'peep-bo'
- bubbles/balloons/picture books
- basic art materials, such as big crayons and washable felt-tip pens.

*Preparation for examination*
- If possible, let the child touch equipment, such as the cassette.

**Pre-school child (2–5 years)**
*Behaviour*
- Take great pride in being able to do things for his- or herself.
- Self-centred: perception of the self as a person.
- Aware of differences between the sexes but this does not affect behaviour.
- Anxiety about ability not to cry under stress (especially boys).
- Play is the most important activity and includes constructive play with other children.
- Begin to comprehend the past/future and today/tomorrow.
- Can reason but lacks logic: fantasy/magic.
- The child often refuses to obey.
- Animistic thinking: all objects are alive.
- Number concept: one, two and many.
- 3–4 years: explanation given in a strange voice is not understood. The same explanation repeated by the parent *is* understood. Therefore communication should be *through* the parent.

### Tips for radiographers

- Use words thoughtfully: cassette, film, bed and dye have different meanings for the child. Do not refer to future surgery as something being 'taken out' or 'cut-off' within the child's hearing.
- Encourage the child and parents to help with positioning. Show how to do it. This may take longer but it is worthwhile.
- Give lots of praise and encouragement.
- Give true answers to the child's questions.
- Do not mistake girls for boys or boys for girls.
- Children like to explore: watch out for safety; they may disappear!

### Anxiety and fears

- Fear that pain will never go away.
- Fear of losing a body part; fear of castration in boys.
- Fear of the dark, solitude and animals.
- Sudden unreasonable fears about objects.
- Increased imagination leads to fantasy fears (shadows).
- Fear that parents will not come back if left alone in the x-ray room.

### Preparation for examination

- show equipment
- explain the procedure to the parents, as before
- focus the child's attention on an imaginary object so as to keep still (a bird in light beam diaphragm (LBD) or a mouse in a corner of the room) for anteroposterior (AP) and lateral skull views
- do not give choices where none exist, such as 'Would you like to come with me?'.

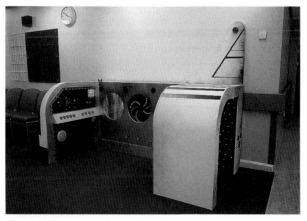

**Figure 1.8a**

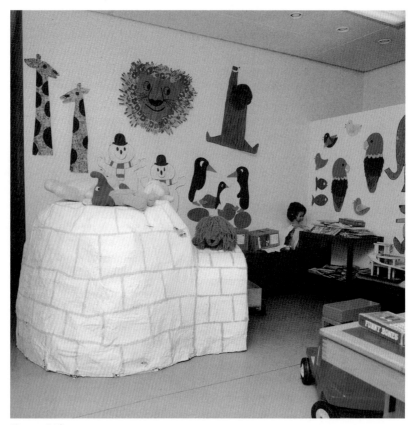

**Figure 1.8b**

*Toys and distractions*
- ◆ bubbles, sand, water, measuring and pouring
- ◆ toys that move/fantasy toys, even a space shuttle in one hospital and an igloo in another (Fig. 1.8a, b)
- ◆ dressing-up clothes, play-house, tea set
- ◆ paper, paints, crayons
- ◆ being read to, singing, finger playing, especially whilst being cuddled by the mother.

### School-age child (5–10 years)

*Behaviour*

- Still needs much reassurance, especially under stress.
- Independent but separation can be stressful; there is anxiety about the ability not to cry under stress (especially boys).
- Advanced motor skills.
- Number concept one to ten (at 5–7 years).
- Can be more aware than able to verbalize.
- Is questioning: he or she watches adults closely, makes assumptions, has a good memory and a rough idea of time intervals.
- Sex differences are important.
- Independent: interaction and socialization are important; friends are more important than family associations.
- Easily hurt, very emotional and has a sense of ethics.
- Can be aggressive and boastful at about 6 years old.

*Tips for radiographers*

- Children may become embarrassed about wanting a parent.
- They understand more than you think: take care what is said in the child's presence.
- It is unwise to say 'Don't worry, it won't hurt.' x-rays do not, but positioning a fractured limb might, and the child will not believe reassurances next time.
- Provide privacy.
- Do not make requests that might embarrass the child in front of other children, e.g. wearing a gown in the waiting room.

*Anxiety and fears*

- Children hate being made fun of or talked down to.
- Anxiety can project into the future: how illness will affect later life.

### Toys and distractions
◆ computer games and videos
◆ board games and building materials, such as glue, scissors, fabric and paint
◆ doll's houses and household items
◆ medical play equipment.

### Preparation for examination
◆ Allay fears that the child might have but is not able to verbalize through not wanting to appear to be a baby.
◆ Let the child lead the conversation by asking open questions.

## Pre-adolescent
### Behaviour
◆ fear/loneliness are often covered up by showing off
◆ age of socialization: peers are most important (at 7–11 years of age)
◆ beginning of ethical sense: right and wrong (at 7–12 years of age)
◆ independent, more self-confident
◆ secondary sexual characteristics may develop or be talked about within groups.

### Tips for radiographers
◆ Be aware that behaviour may be attention seeking; set limits and stick to them.
◆ Reassure without being patronizing.
◆ Building trust is important.
◆ Allow some choices, for instance 'Do you want your mum/dad to come in with you?'.
◆ Respect privacy.

### Anxiety and fears
◆ Being made to feel foolish, especially in front of peers.
◆ Having nothing to do: being bored can raise anxiety levels.

### Toys and distractions
◆ magazines, comics and books
◆ pens, paint, paper, doodle art
◆ computer games and videos.

### Preparation for examination
◆ Give honest information in an environment where all involved can ask questions openly (child patient and parents).
◆ Use actual equipment to show what will happen.
◆ Reassure the child that fear and tears are perfectly normal.

### Adolescent (13–16 years)

*Behaviour*
- Detachment from family; is independent but may not like being away from friends and peer groups; may be antagonistic towards adults.
- May have developed sexual relationships and may be sexually active.
- Will be extremely aware of physical changes; body image will be linked to self-esteem and acceptance by peers. There will be growth spurts and the patient will be emotionally vulnerable and self-conscious, and possibly clumsy, embarrassed and shy.
- Apathy and negativity may be a cover for true feelings.
- A teenager the capacity for abstract thought, is idealistic, sees issues in 'black and white' and has dogmatic opinions.

*Tips for radiographers*
- The adolescent may still need a parent when under stress.
- Do not impose your own moral values.
- Provide privacy and respect; treat as an adult.
- Show that you understand how they are feeling.
- Do not expect adolescents to always behave like adults; rebellious, testing behaviour may be a response to fear or anger.

*Anxiety and fears*
- being treated like a child
- being forced to participate.

*Distractions*
- computers/TV/video/stereo
- magazines aimed at this age group
- electronic games
- playing cards and gadgets.

*Preparation for examination*
- Give honest explanations, encouraging trust.
- Ensure that explanations are understood; the adolescent patient may have a fear of appearing 'stupid' and might not ask questions.
- Ensure that parents are included in the preparation; it is easy to overlook them in this age group.

**Language**
- Children's vocabulary is appropriate to their concepts.
- A complete system of communication exists at each stage.
- Language is an unfolding process controlled by maturation.

### First year
- One word sentences, e.g. 'Teddy' equals 'This is Teddy', 'I want Teddy', 'Where is Teddy?'.

- One word for many types, such as 'Dog' for all four-legged furry animals.

- Realization grows gradually of differences in:
  - type: new words such as cow or horse
  - situation: dog in a book, on TV, as a toy or as a live pet.

### Second year
- Two-word sentences, such as 'Mummy shoe', 'Teddy up', 'Drink milk', 'No bed'.

- A growing understanding of events happening and relationship between things.

- Refers to self by name – 'Joseph do'.

- 'Telegram'-type conversation continues till approximately 3 to 4 years of age.

### Third year
- Learning new names: 'What is...?'.

- Refers to self as I, not by own name.

### Fourth year
- Asks 'How, why?' questions.

- Talks in sentences.

Many 'hospital' words are not understood even by schoolchildren (such as barium; abdomen) or they may have a different meaning (theatre; film; sucker).

The thoughtful use of words is essential when explanations are given such as dye or cuts (as in computerized tomography). 'Take a photograph of your insides' can also sound threatening.

Explanations given in unfamiliar voices may not be understood, while the same explanations given by parents are. Therefore communication should be through the parents.

- Sick children are an enormous strain on parents and families.

**Parents**
- There is a need to involve the parents in x-ray examinations.

- In modern nursing, parents are crucial in the child's care. Some radiology departments do not encourage parents to stay with their child, or even try to exclude them. The parents should be encouraged to stay – the child needs the parents' emotional support.

**Staff**  Radiographers need to be trained in:

- how to communicate with children
- how to deal with difficult situations
- child psychology
- strategies to deal with unhelpful/uncooperative parents
- how to avoid making difficult situations worse, for instance parents asking for gonad protection for their child when it is unnecessary and the radiographer replies 'I know my job, you don't have to tell me'.

Essential qualities of a good paediatric radiographer are as follows:

- understands and is able to empathize with the needs of the child and family
- experienced, appropriately trained and able to gain the confidence of the child and parents/carers
- friendly, smiling, has sense of humour, innovative and enthusiastic
- wants to work with children
- not upset or disturbed by sick children
- not judgemental of the family situations.

**Play**  'Play as a concept is exceptionally difficult to define but it has come to be recognized as a normal and essential requirement for a child's well-being and development.' (From *Hospital, a deprived environment for children*, Save the Children Fund Report, 1989)

Radiology departments should recognize the great advantage of consulting a play specialist. Departmental budgets rarely allow for this but there may well be one available within the hospital.

***Benefits of play for the radiographer***

- Play aids normality for the child patient and family.
- Reduces stress and anxiety for child, parents and the radiographer.
- It facilitates communication between the radiographer and the child/family.
- Aids preparation for radiographic procedures.
- Improves staff/child/family relationships.
- It is fun; it is worthwhile spending a little time because of improved results.

**The role of the play specialist**

■ To teach the value of play and put it on the agenda.

■ Designing methods of play preparation for procedures.

■ Helping to create a child-friendly environment.

■ Supporting families, including parents and siblings.

■ Working as part of a multidisciplinary team within the radiology department.

**Types of play**

■ Toys and distractions should be targeted at each stage of psychological and physical development (as listed previously).

■ A child-centred environment should include appropriate play for babies, toddlers, school-age children and adolescents:
  ● a soft, safe play area for babies
  ● drawing, colouring, painting and crafts
  ● a playing house and construction toys
  ● board games, crosswords and word search puzzles
  ● magazines and books
  ● 'doctors and nurses' play
  ● puppets/bubbles
  ● computer and video games; music
  ● interactive games such as table football
  ● pets: Pets as Therapy (PAT).

**Play preparation**

■ Play can be used to prepare for, or minimize, the frightening aspects of radiographic examinations.

■ Information should be given from a child's point of view.

■ There should be an awareness that children might still react adversely, even after play preparation; it may need more than one session to be successful.

*WARNING*  If play is not carried out properly it can increase anxiety.

■ Preparation should be carried out in stages:
  ● establish what the child and parents know and their previous experiences
  ● obtain permission from parents
  ● correct any misconceptions
  ● decide on preparation or distractions
  ● encourage questions from the child; inform other relevant staff of your decisions.

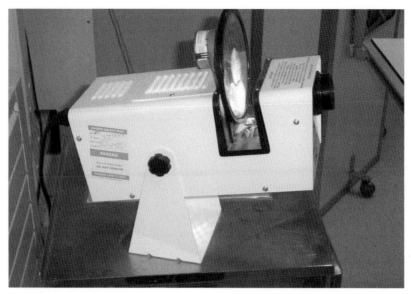

**Figure 1.9**

**Distraction**  Distraction is used to help a child cope with unpleasant, strange and unfamiliar situations, including x-ray examinations.

Children who are helped to cope with painful procedures learn methods of coping that can be applied to other stressful situations including hospital examinations and visits to the dentist.
Distraction:

- gives a child the opportunity for choice, control and involvement
- the key is the interaction between the child, parents and radiographer
- calming is extremely beneficial to staff as well as the child
- the child must be praised
- does not always work.

**Distraction techniques**

- stroking; nursery rhymes; dummy/pacifier
- bubble blowing/bubble-making machine
- music boxes, musical toys and books, and music tapes
- projector (Fig. 1.9) and mobiles
- puppets
- encouraging the child to bring a favourite toy or music tape
- counting devices, such as beads on an abacus
- singing
- recounting favourite things or places
- joke telling
- guided imagery.

# 2 Radiation protection and immobilization

**Radiation protection**

- Radiation risk is dependent on the age at which the child is exposed. Exposure before the age of 10 years results in risks of genetic effects and leukaemia that are 4–7 times greater than in adults.

- Many radiographic examinations are not necessary. Article 3 of the *Ionising Radiations (Medical Exposures) Regulations* (HMSO, 2000) requires that all exposures should be justified, ensuring that there is a net benefit to the individual who is to be exposed to offset the detriment associated with ionizing radiation. Ensuring that only those examinations that have a direct effect on patient management are carried out considerably reduces exposure to radiation.

- Request forms should be signed by an appropriate referrer, have adequate clinical information and meet agreed referral criteria. Examinations must be justified and relevant. If the clinical question can be answered by an alternative imaging technique which does not involve ionizing radiation, that should be the preferred option, if available.

- The most important factors for minimizing the radiation dose are:
  - Employing high speed film/screen combinations.
  - High kV and short exposure times.
  - Avoid using antiscatter grids whenever possible. The omission of a grid/Potter–Bucky for X-ray examinations of the skull, abdomen and hips is worth considering. A small child produces so little scatter that the reduction in image quality through not using a grid does not reduce the amount of useful information but it does halve the radiation dose. (R Nicholson, Radiation Protection Advisor and Clinical Physicist, St Mary's Hospital, Paddington, London, pers. comm.)
  - Tight collimation with light beam diaphragm (LBD) edges visible on X-ray film.
  - Low attenuation materials must be used, such as carbon fibre tabletops.
  - Lead gonad protection, which is the correct size and shape, should be applied whenever possible. Care should also be taken to shield the developing breast and thyroid, both of which are radiosensitive. Lead rubber shielding over areas of the body next to the primary beam can reduce the dose by up to 40%. A variety of commercial lead gonad protection is available in many shapes and sizes (Fig. 2.1).

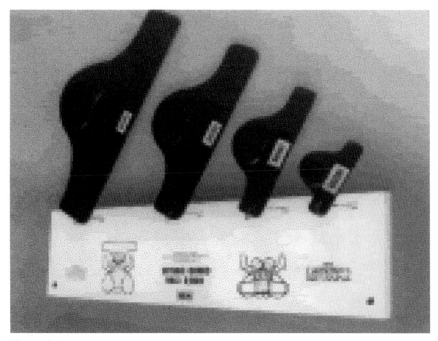

Figure 2.1a

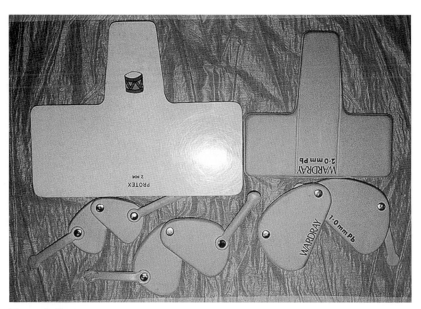

Figure 2.1b

- Lead rubber should always be placed on top of incubators in neonatal work.
- The breasts and sternum must be protected when the abdomen is X-rayed.
- Additional tube filtration of the primary beam should be used to absorb unnecessary soft radiation and reduce patient dose.
- Dose area product meters should be used and dosimetry performed regularly.
- Protection must be used for holders. Lead aprons of all sizes, including child size and half aprons (Fig. 2.2 a,b). Screens are useful for siblings or helpers to distract the child (Fig. 2.3).

## Immobilization

■ The smaller size of children, and their faster heart and respiratory rates contribute to movement blur in addition to their sometimes being uncooperative. Therefore good quality images may be difficult to produce.

■ Immobilization devices are available but they can seem horrific from a child's perspective (see Chapter 1, pages 1 and 3) and might cause emotional disturbances and a life-long fear of hospitals.

■ Understanding children's needs, providing a child-friendly environment and well-trained staff (see Chapter 1) ensures high-quality images and can eliminate the use of most immobilization aids (Fig. 2.4).

■ To avoid mechanical immobilization:
  - The examination must be performed quickly and accurately.
  - Everything must be ready beforehand, exposure set, orientation markers, correct size of film, tube position and protection.
  - Use the shortest possible exposure times.
  - Use fast film/screen combinations.
  - The child should be as comfortable as possible.
  - Use innovative positioning, for instance the hand is easier to X-ray if the child is prone (see Fig. 8.63, p. 167).

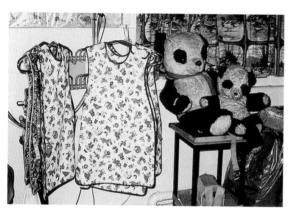

Figure 2.2a

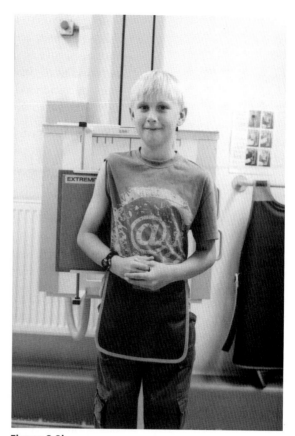

Figure 2.2b

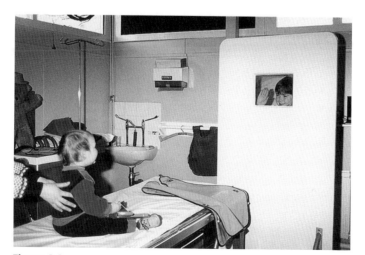

Figure 2.3

■ Simple aids such as Velcro, Dycem, sandbags and foam pads (including child skull pad) can be used to aid immobilization. Bucky bands (which have been sold as standard table accessories until recently and can often be found in the back of X-ray room cupboards) provide an invaluable immobilization aid. Mechanical or physical restraint should be used only with parental consent (see Chapter 10, pages 220 and 221).

■ If immobilization is necessary this should be done with as little upset to the child and parents as possible.

■ Incorrect positioning and bad holding techniques are often the cause of inadequate imaging.

**Pregnancy question**

■ The *Ionising Radiations (Medical Exposure) Regulations* (HMSO, 2000) require that, when a female of reproductive age presents for an examination in which the primary beam irradiates the pelvic area, she should be asked whether she is/might be pregnant.

■ Parents/patients should be warned before they arrive in the department that all patients who are of reproductive age and who are having an examination involving irradiating the pelvis will be asked about the possibility of pregnancy.

■ Note that the patient may deny pregnancy (or the possibility of pregnancy) if asked when a parent is present but may admit the possibility to the radiographer in confidence. Departments should have policies in place to help the radiographer in dilemmas about confidentiality.

■ When there is a doubt about the possibility of pregnancy, the examination may either be postponed until a later date or carried out if clinically urgent. This decision has to be made by the referrer or consultant radiologist.

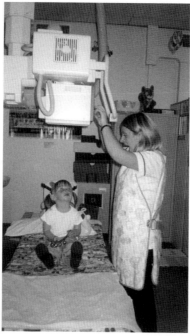

**Figure 2.4**

***Computed (digital) radiography (CR)***

Specific problems with children include:

■ Lack of collimation marks on the image.

■ The incorrect choice of cassette size and inaccurate positioning on the plate; careful positioning is required with the area of interest in the centre of the cassette. Exposures should be made symmetrically on the cassette with no overlap of the collimated field.

■ Only small areas of the cassette may be used in some cases, e.g. an X-ray image collimated to a baby's finger. CR requires a third of the plate to be covered.

■ The inability to check the radiation dose. Overexposure will produce beautiful images and underexposure will appear grainy, therefore there is a tendency to overexpose.

■ Shuttering, post-processing, gives the appearance of a well-collimated field but this may not be the same as the actual field. As digital shuttering can mask the lack of correct collimation of the X-ray beam there is no visible record of how much the child may have been irradiated unnecessarily. This is particularly important when imaging neonates as the accumulated radiation dose from possibly daily radiographs in the first weeks of life needs consideration, especially as the dose is not reduced by digital technology (contrary to widespread belief).

Although CR slightly increases the dose for each exposure, repeat films are not needed as the image can be manipulated post-processing. Therefore the radiation dose overall is likely to be reduced.

# 3 The chest

**Positioning**

■ Usually supine until the child can sit up unaided (about 6 months of age) (Figs 3.1, 3.2).

■ Usually anteroposterior (AP) projection until 3 or 4 years old (Figs 3.3–3.5).

■ A lateral view is taken only if requested by a consultant radiologist or radiographer practitioner.

■ Accuracy is essential. The younger or smaller the child, the greater the chance of misleading appearances from inexact positioning.

■ Main positioning points:
  ● head kept straight between arms (Figs 3.3, 3.5)
  ● if supine, the adult should hold the baby's forearms (Fig. 3.2)
  ● if erect, the arms are held against the sides of the head with elbows flexed pointing forwards (Figs 3.3, 3.5)
  ● 2–5 year olds are better sitting rather than standing (Fig. 3.6)

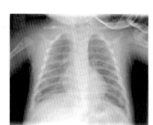

Figure 3.1

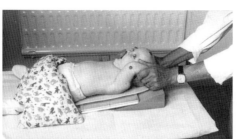

Figure 3.2

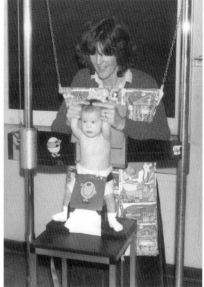

Figure 3.3

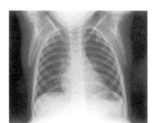

Figure 3.4

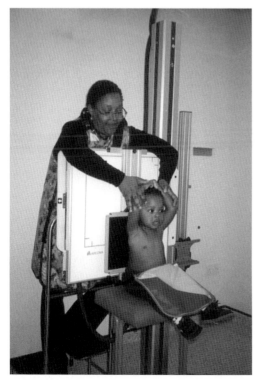

Figure 3.5

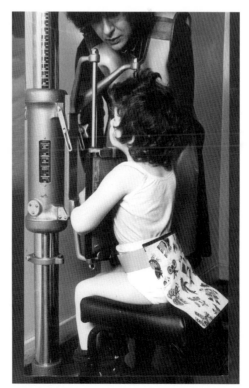

Figure 3.6

- children aged 5 years and over can stand for a posteroanterior (PA) projection with the arms around the cassette or holding onto the erect Bucky (Figs 3.7–3.9).

■ Radiation dose to adult's hands: Figures 3.2 and 3.3, 0.002 mSv maximum (Gyll and Blake, 1986).

*Discussion*
■ Some kind of seat with Velcro straps attached is essential if under 5s are to be x-rayed erect. The design of the seat in Fig. 3.3 has been described (Gyll, 1983).

■ Different methods of holding, which are equally valid, have evolved in various children's hospitals.

■ Immobilization devices are commercially available (Pig-o-Stat, etc.). Disadvantages of these are:
  - over-inflated lungs from inevitable crying
  - longterm emotional damage (see Chapter 1).

**Radiation protection**
■ The primary beam must be collimated within the area of the cassette.

■ Paediatric lead rubber aprons, obtainable in several sizes, should be used for gonad protection.

■ The child's thyroid should not be within the primary beam field. This should be achieved through accurate collimation (it may not be possible with babies).

■ An adult holding the child from behind a chest-stand must be protected by a screen or lead rubber coat of not less than 0.5 mm lead equivalent.

■ The adult's hands must be outside the primary beam.

■ Scattered dose is negligible; gloves may impede correct holding.

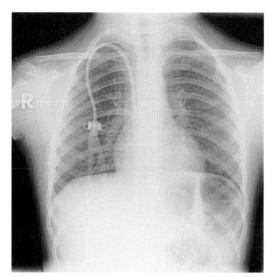

Figure 3.7

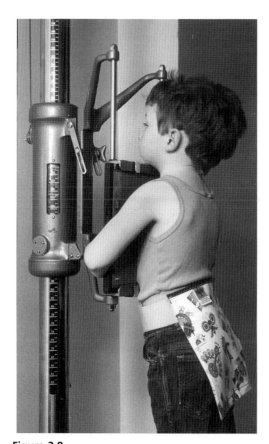

Figure 3.8

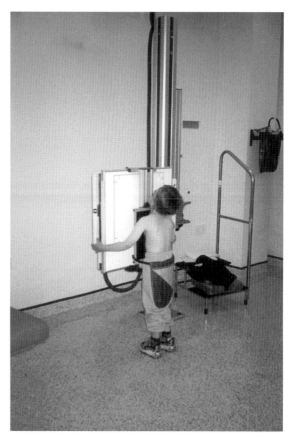

Figure 3.9

**Technical points**

■ Cassette sizes are not based on human anatomy. Up to 7 or 8 years old the cassette is used crosswise rather than upright, as this matches the shape of the chest better (Fig. 3.10).

■ Using the cassette upright can cause over-irradiation by the unintended inclusion of the upper abdomen (Fig. 3.11). Also, the namespace may overlie the lung apex (Fig. 3.12a). The child may move on inspiration (Fig. 3.12b): a 30 cm × 40 cm (15 in × 12 in) cassette should have been used in both cases.

■ Recommended cassette sizes:
18 cm × 24 cm (10 in × 8 in) up to 9 to 12 months
24 cm × 30 cm (10 in × 12 in) 1 to 7 or 8 years
30 cm × 40 cm (12 in × 15 in) over 8 years, but collimate the lower third of the film out of the x-ray field.

■ The edges of the radiation field should be seen inside the film edges.

■ The shortest possible exposure time is required, therefore a high-output generator is needed including mobiles.

■ If follow-up radiography is likely, exposure factors and projections must be the same as for the first examination.

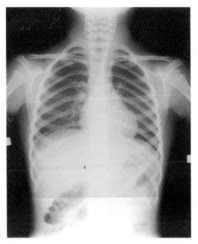

Figure 3.10

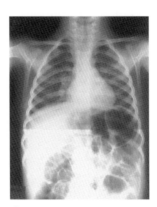

Figure 3.11a

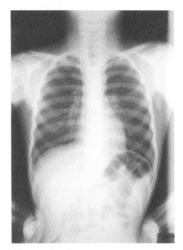

Figure 3.11b

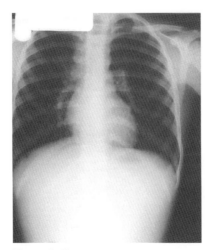

Figure 3.12a

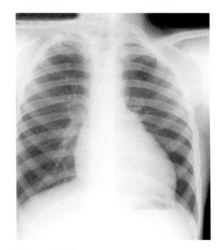

Figure 3.12b

**Common faults**

The three main faults are rotation, lordosis and expiration. All three of these alter the size and/or shape of the heart and hilum, and cause differences in lung translucency.

*Rotation*

**Criteria**

- The length of the anterior rib ends should be equal.

- The medial clavicle end should be symmetrical to the sternum; notice how the arms have been held.

**Cause**

Turned head because the child is held only by the arms (Figs 3.13, 3.14). NOTE The adult's hands have been irradiated (Fig. 3.13b).

**Correction**

The child's head is held **between** the arms (Figs 3.2, 3.3, 3.5, 3.6).

*NOTE*   Even if held correctly, the effect of very slight rotation is seen in Fig. 3.15a: there is a difference in lung translucency. This is corrected in a repeat radiograph (Fig. 3.15b).

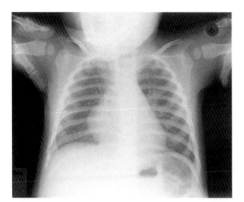

Figure 3.13a

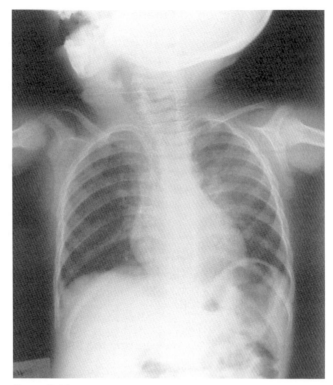

Figure 3.14

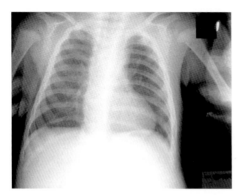

Figure 3.13b

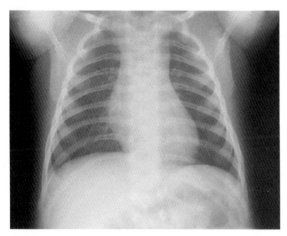

Figure 3.15a

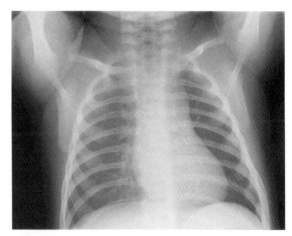

Figure 3.15b

## *Lordotic projection*

### Criteria

■ The anterior rib ends should be below the posterior rib ends, not parallel to or above them as in Fig. 3.16.

■ The medial ends of the clavicles should be below the first or second ribs.

### Causes

■ If a baby's or toddler's back is parallel to the cassette with the x-ray beam at right angles, the projection will be lordotic:
- supine baby lying flat on cassette
- holder pulling erect baby flat back against the cassette
- baby sitting in a 'slumped' position with legs extended at the same level (Fig. 3.17a).

■ Arms extended straight above the head, supine or erect, makes the child lean back

■ Child arching back, away from the cassette in the PA position

■ Centring too low.

### Correction

■ 15° foam pad in the supine position (Fig. 3.2) and behind the head or shoulders in the AP erect position, see Fig. 3.17b (see also Fig. 3.3). NOTE Tube angulation may be used instead of a foam pad but the x-ray field must be contained within the film edges.

■ The baby's legs should be lower than his or her bottom, i.e. the baby is sitting upright on a foam pad or similar (Fig. 3.17b).

■ Arms held with the elbows flexed (see Fig. 3.3).

Figure 3.18 shows (a) the shape of the baby's chest: extended legs cause the protruding abdomen to tilt the chest backwards, (b) inevitable lordotic projection with horizontal beam and (c) corrected position with 15° foam pad behind the shoulders.

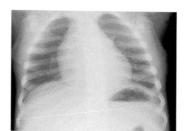

Figure 3.16

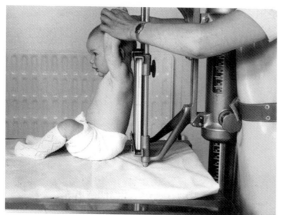

Figure 3.17a

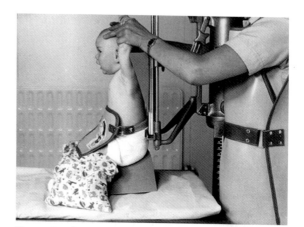

Figure 3.17b

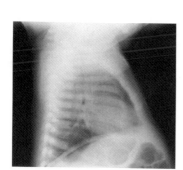

Figure 3.18a

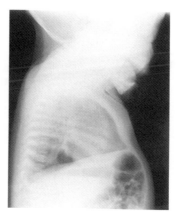

Figure 3.18b

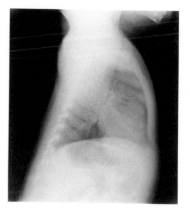

Figure 3.18c

*Expiration*

### Criterion

Nine posterior or five anterior ribs should be seen above the diaphragm. The film shown in Fig. 3.19 is unacceptable.

### Cause

Mistiming the exposure.

### Correction

- If the child is too young to cooperate, expose on full inspiration, during normal respiration.

- Babies' and toddlers' breathing is abdominal: watch for an expanded abdomen in the AP position. If positioned PA, watch for a sideways bulge of the abdomen below ribcage.

- Rehearse an older child: 'Breathe in and hold breath'. If this is difficult for the child, ask to 'Breathe in' and expose at peak inspiration.

- Watch that the child's shoulders do not rise on breathing in.

### Note

- **The child/baby must not be crying during exposure.** If so, inspiration will be too deep, causing over-inflated lungs giving misleading appearances which can be mistaken for pathology.

- The differences in appearances on inspiration/expiration are more marked than in adults (Figs 3.20, 2 months old; 3.21, 4 years old).

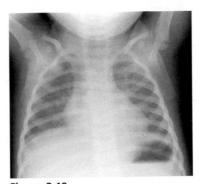

**Figure 3.19**

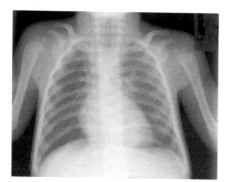

Figure 3.20a

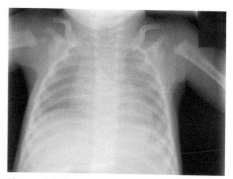

Figure 3.20b

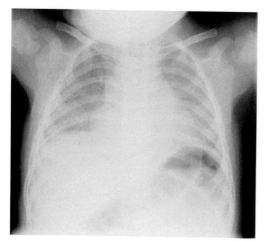

Figure 3.21a

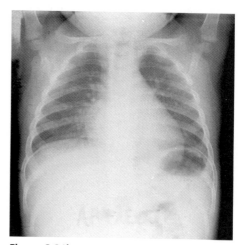

Figure 3.21b

**Exposure factors**

- Time factor must not be more than 0.01 seconds.

- The same exposure factors must be used for follow-up films. They should be noted on the first examination and referred to by the radiographer/technologist on subsequent examinations. Otherwise the films will not be comparable (Figs 3.22a,b) even though taken on the same degree of inspiration.

- Automatic exposure controls (AEC) should not be used.

- Chronic asthmatics may need less exposure if emphysema is present (Fig. 3.23).

- If a request for a lateral view of any condition is approved, the necessary increase in exposure is less than for an adult, only 15–20 kV.

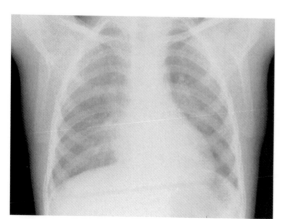

Figure 3.22a

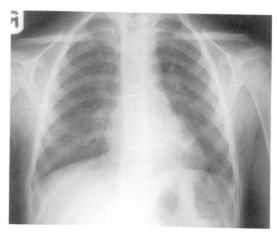

Figure 3.22b

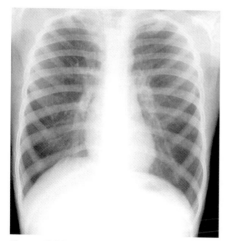

Figure 3.23

**Artefacts**

- A misplaced 15° foam pad can cause a projection of the soft tissues of the face over the apices (Fig. 3.24).

- Clothing, even if cotton, may be seen over the lungs. Vest on a 6-year-old (Fig. 3.25a) and on a 13-year-old (Fig. 3.25b). Plasticized printing on T-shirts is radiopaque.

- Long hair plait left hanging down the child's back; should be pinned up on the head (Fig. 3.26).

- Bobble holding hair in a ponytail (Fig. 3.27).

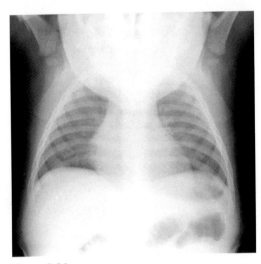

**Figure 3.24**

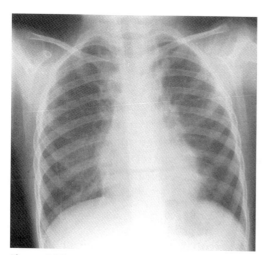

Figure 3.25a

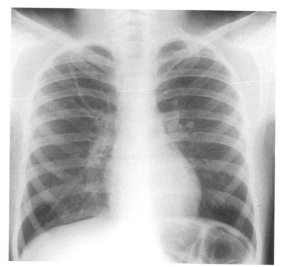

Figure 3.25b

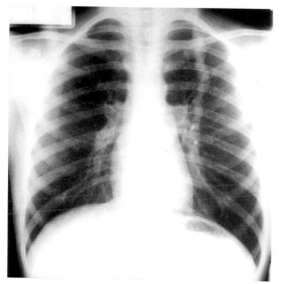

Figure 3.26

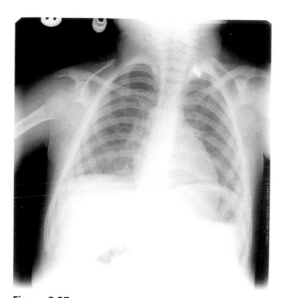

Figure 3.27

**Pathology needing extra views**

- Two kinds, both present with symptomatic stridor:
  - acute laryngotracheitis 6 months to 3 years approximately
  - acute epiglottitis 2 to 7 years of age approximately.

*Croup*

- Both conditions require AP erect chest and lateral view of the neck (Fig. 3.28).

- Acute epiglottitis is severe and can be life threatening. The child must not be upset or caused to struggle, as either may result in crying, choking and respiratory arrest. **Do not position supine as this may cause complete airway obstruction. No matter how ill, the child must always be x-rayed in the erect AP position.**

- There must be a qualified nurse with the child, and a doctor immediately available for intubation if needed.

*Inhaled foreign body (FB)*

- Inspiration/expiration films are essential, even on a young child who is unable to co-operate. **Films must be taken erect to avoid the possibility of complete airway obstruction.**

- **The child must not be upset or struggle as total airway obstruction may result.**

- Figure 3.29 shows an inhaled peanut in a 13-month-old child: partial obstruction of the left bronchus – obstructive emphysema. Fig. 3.29 (a) shows inspiration and (b) expiration.

- Figure 3.30. Inhaled peanut in a 3-year-old child: complete obstruction of the left bronchus, collapsed lung (atelectasis). (a) Evening, diagnosis missed in A & E; (b) next morning: emergency bronchoscopy saved the child's life.

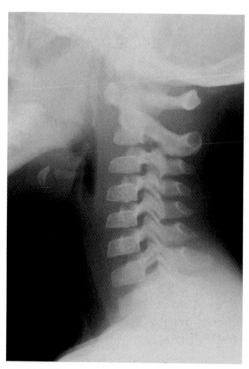

Figure 3.28

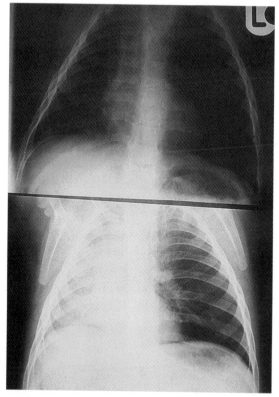

Figure 3.29a,b

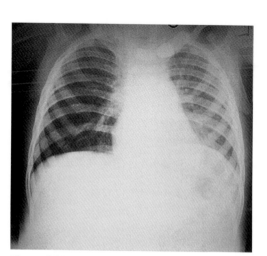

Figure 3.30a

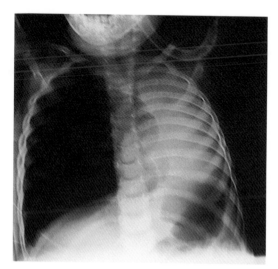

Figure 3.30b

# 4 The abdomen

Ultrasound is the first choice of imaging for obstruction, perforation, etc. An anteroposterior (AP) supine view may also be needed as well (Fig. 4.1: a, 2 months old; b, 1 year old; c, 5 years old). Positioning for erect, decubitus and lateral views is included for use when an experienced paediatric sonographer is not available, e.g. out of hours, in primary care centres or in remote locations.

**Positioning (supine)**

- Younger children's legs are immobilized with a Bucky band and foam pad (Fig. 4.2).

- The assisting parent should stand at the head of the table (not at the side) to ensure that the child lies straight (Fig. 4.2). Adult hands, which are distant from the x-ray beam, do not need lead gloves.

- An older child can lie without being held. Note the pants' elastic at the symphysis pubis and gonad protection (lead rubber apron).

**Technical points**

- An instruction to hold the breath out (as adults are instructed) is confusing. The cooperative child should be told to 'Take a small breath in, stop breathing'. This should be rehearsed before the exposure is made. Babies' and toddlers' breathing is abdominal. The rise (inspiration) and fall (expiration) of the abdomen should be watched and exposure made on expiration, when there is a slight pause.

- A child's abdomen is two-thirds of the total body length. Collimate from the level of the nipples to the symphysis pubis. The cassette used should be large enough for the nameplate to be outside of the abdominal area. There is a tendency to collimate the diaphragm off.

- Gonad protection should always be used on boys (Fig. 4.2b; see also Fig. 4.12, p. 59).

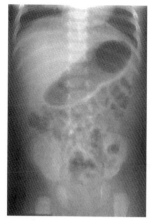

Figure 4.1a

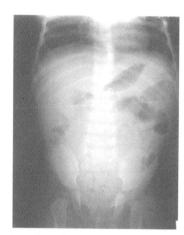

Figure 4.1b

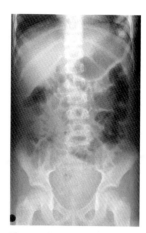

Figure 4.1c

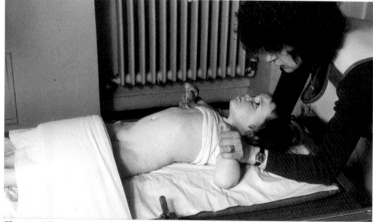

Figure 4.2a

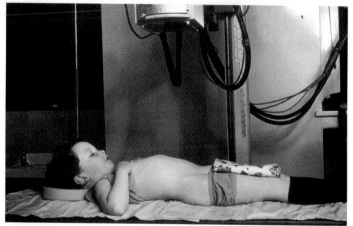

Figure 4.2b

■ Use of the Potter–Bucky grid makes accurate positioning easier; omitting it reduces the radiation dose.

■ Correct sizes for approximate age ranges:
- 18 cm × 24 cm (10 in × 8 in) up to 6 months old
- 24 cm × 30 cm (12 in × 10 in) from 6 months to 3 or 4 years
- 30 cm × 40 cm (15 in × 12 in) from 4 to 9 or 10 years
- 35 cm × 43 cm (17 in × 14 in) for 9 or 10 years and above.

***Common faults*** ■ Too small a film (Figs 4.3 and 4.4).

■ Figure 4.3:
(a) a 7-year-old on 24 cm × 30 cm film (12 in × 10 in);
(b) a 10-year-old on 24 cm × 30 cm film (12 in × 10 in);
(c) a 13-year-old on 30 cm × 40 cm film (15 in × 12 in); and
(d) shows the 13-year-old's abdomen on the correct size of film.

■ Too small a film and inaccurate centring because the child (3 months of age) was laid directly on the 18 × 24 cm cassette (Fig. 4.4a).

■ 24 × 30 cm cassette in a Potter–Bucky tray enables accurate positioning and collimation (Fig. 4.4b).

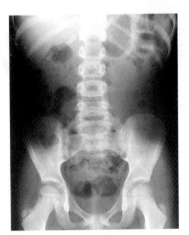

Figure 4.3a

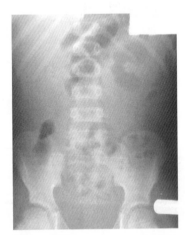

Figure 4.3b

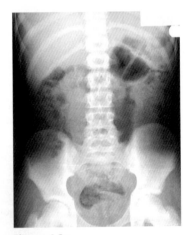

Figure 4.3c

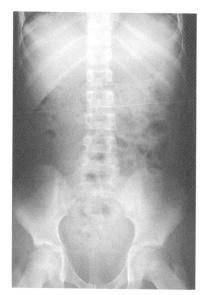

Figure 4.3d

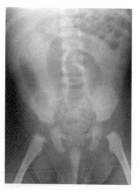

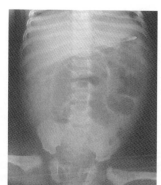

Figure 4.4a                    Figure 4.4b

■ The abdomen of a baby or toddler (Fig. 4.5) is a different shape from that of the older child (Fig. 4.6, 8 years old).

■ Lateral collimation, as for an adult, excludes part of the child's abdominal organs; the abdominal contents go right to edge of abdomen as there is no fat layer.

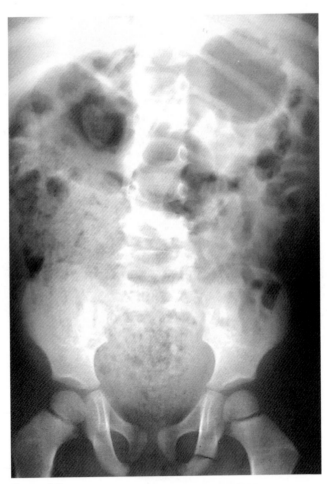

**Figure 4.5**

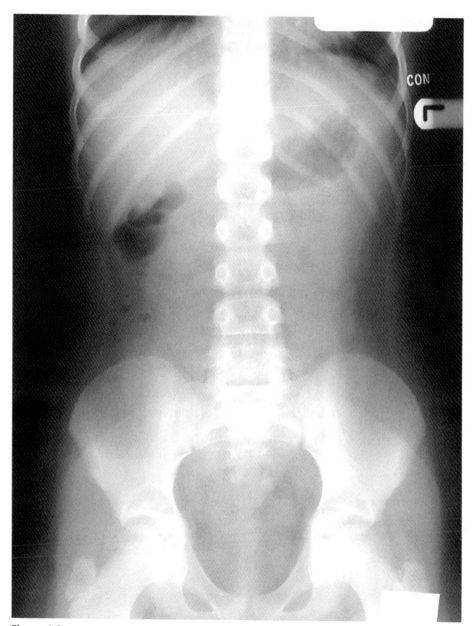

Figure 4.6

**Positioning (erect)**

■ Ultrasound is the first choice of imaging for obstruction, perforation, etc. If ultrasound is not readily available, an erect AP view should be taken only when requested by an agreed authority. In the UK this will be a radiographic practitioner – as defined in the *Ionising Radiations (Medical Exposures) Regulations* – but elsewhere it would probably be a consultant radiologist or surgeon.

■ It is essential to sit the baby/toddler/young child on some kind of seat so that the legs are lower than the abdomen. Figure 4.7 shows a specially made seat for chest and erect abdomen radiography.

■ Figure 4.8 shows improvisations if a seat is not available.
  ● standard chest-stand at table end, 45° foam pad and sandbags (Fig. 4.8a)
  ● polystyrene box as seat, Velcro strap around box and legs, cassette taped to step on fluoroscopy table (Fig. 4.8b).

■ An older child could sit on a rectangular foam pad on a stool so that the legs are lower. If well enough the child could stand (Fig. 4.9).

■ A baby's arms should be held up beside the head. The dose to unprotected adult hands in Figs 4.7 and 4.8 is not more than 0.005 mSv (Gyll and Blake, 1986).

■ The whole abdomen should be included. There is a tendency to collimate the rectum off, or obscure it with lead.

■ A child-sized lead apron can be used for gonad protection and immobilization if the straps are long enough to go around the cassette as well as the child (Fig. 4.9).

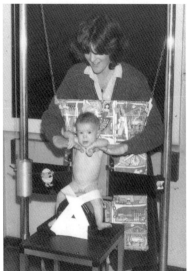

Figure 4.7

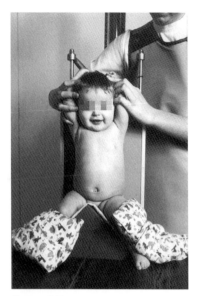

Figure 4.8a

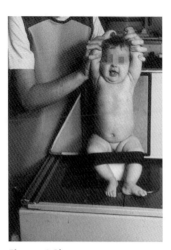

Figure 4.8b

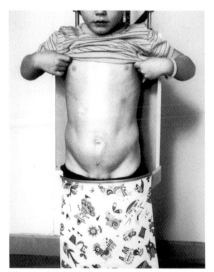

Figure 4.9

**Technical points**    Breath-holding instructions and expiration estimate, as for supine position.

**Common faults**    ■ Inadequate positioning, such as leaving the legs on the same level as the buttocks. In Fig. 4.10 the babies are probably sitting on the x-ray table with the cassette propped or held behind: (a) 3 months old; (b) 6 months old. Accurate positioning is impossible.

■ The rectum is often collimated off (Fig. 4.11a) or obscured by misplaced gonad protection (Fig. 4.11b). Unless positioning is accurate, adequate collimation is extremely difficult; a large area of the chest is often mistakenly included.

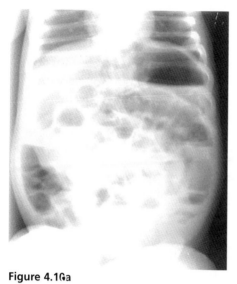

Figure 4.10a

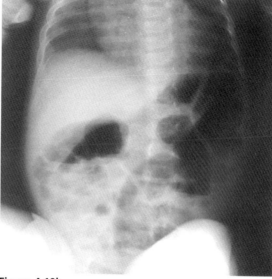

Figure 4.10b

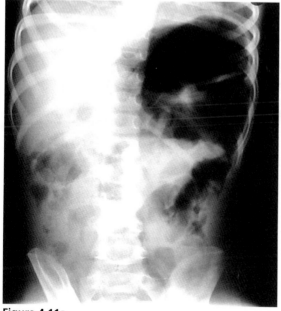

Figure 4.11a

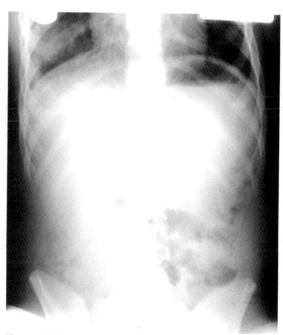

Figure 4.11b

**Positioning (decubitus)**

■ If an older child is too ill to stand, decubitus positioning is used. The word 'decubitus' means 'lying down': it is frequently misunderstood and misused.

■ The lateral decubitus position with horizontal beam projection gives an AP or PA view (Fig. 4.12a). Dorsal decubitus positioning with horizontal beam projection gives a lateral view. 'Lateral decubitus' refers only to the patient's position, not the radiographic view. 'Horizontal beam lateral' (often abbreviated to HBL) has been seen written on an AP view!

■ The position for a lateral decubitus horizontal beam PA view is shown in Fig. 4.12b. Note the use of lead rubber for gonad protection.

■ Position for a lateral view of 1-year-old's abdomen with vertical beam projection: shoulders held by an adult, hips held lateral by two 45° foam pads, one each side, under a Bucky band (Fig. 4.13).

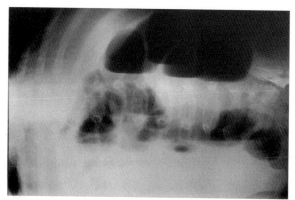

Figure 4.12a

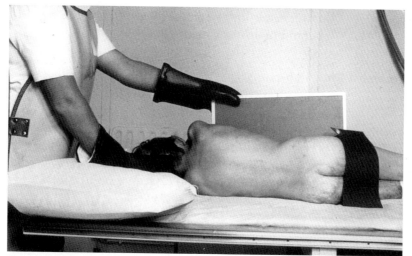

Figure 4.12b

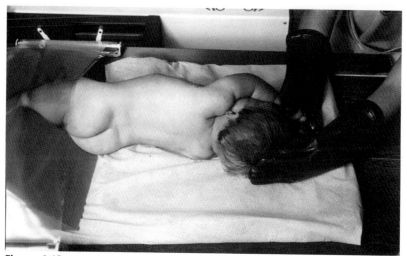

Figure 4.13

## Swallowed foreign bodies

### Discussion

- Several recent studies have queried the practice of routine x-ray examination for all swallowed foreign bodies (FBs).

- Small, round, smooth objects, such as coins (Fig. 4.14), almost invariably travel safely through the gastrointestinal tract. Routine delayed films are not justifiable.

- Long, thin or sharp FB, such as hairgrips, may become impacted in the duodenum (Fig. 4.15).

- 'Button' batteries need x-raying to monitor their progress and integrity because of the danger of mercury poisoning (Fig. 4.16).

- Metal detectors are used in some A & E departments instead of radiography, avoiding irradiation (Tidey, 1995). These can also locate metals of low radiodensity such as the ring pull of an aluminium drinks can.

### Positioning

The child is undressed and lies supine with the head turned to one side to demonstrate the pharynx (Fig. 4.17).

### Technical points

- The approximate time of swallowing should be noted. If within the previous 12 hours, the film should include the neck, chest and abdomen to iliac crests only, excluding the gonads (Fig. 4.17). A 35 cm × 43 cm (17 in × 14 in) cassette is needed for a 4 to 5-year-old child.

- Under 2 or 3 years old, omit the Potter–Bucky grid (less radiation).

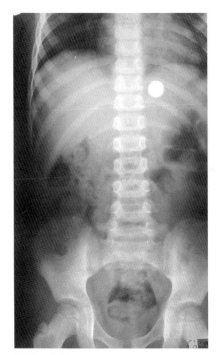

Figure 4.14

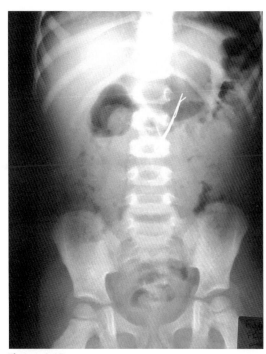

Figure 4.15

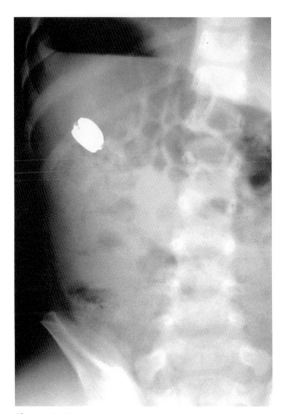

Figure 4.16

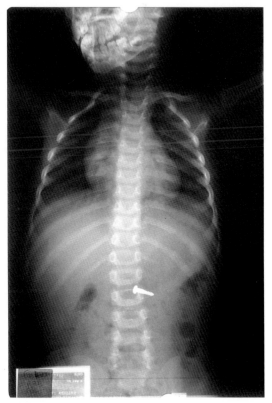

Figure 4.17

- If the parent brings an example of the FB that has been swallowed, such as beads from a broken necklace or piece of a toy, it should be x-rayed to check its opacity. Glass may be opaque: Fig. 4.18 shows (a) a wineglass with a piece bitten out by a 7-month-old baby; (b) the swallowed glass fragment.

- Upper oesophageal FB in a young child, less than 2 years of age, can present as stridor. Figure 4.19 shows the chest film of a 6-month-old baby with stridor (whose twin brother had whooping cough) showing a totally unsuspected coin in the oesophagus.

- Over approximately 5 to 6 years old, two cassettes are needed. If the abdomen is x-rayed first and a FB seen, the second film can be omitted, hence lessening the radiation dose.

- If no FB is seen on the abdominal film, a PA oblique view (erect) of the mediastinum and pharynx is preferable to a standard chest x-ray.

- If a confirmed oesophageal FB is to be removed under general anaesthetic, a second film should be taken immediately beforehand to check if the FB has passed into the stomach.

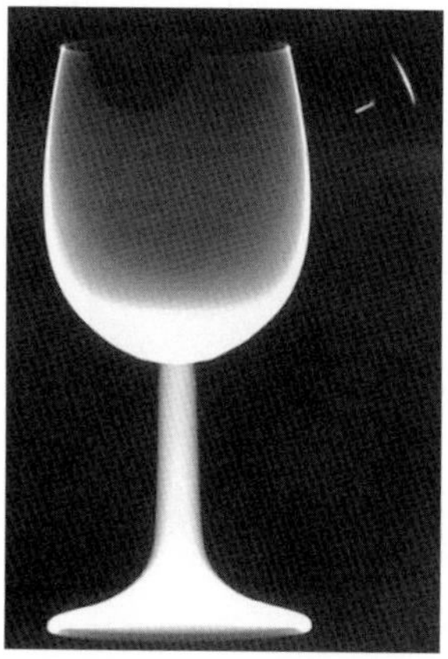

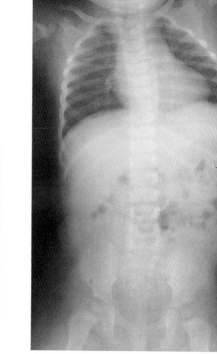

Figure 4.18b

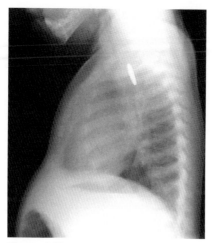

Figure 4.18a

Figure 4.19

***Common faults***
- Omitting to undress the child (Figs 4.20, 4.21). Opacity apparently in the oesophagus in Fig. 4.20, which was thought to be related to a screw in the stomach, is in fact the zip on a 3-year-old's dress.

- Figure 4.21: (a) was taken with the child's cotton T-shirt left on; (b) was taken after the removal of the T-shirt and chain. The 'medal' is in the oesophagus.

- The pharynx not included when a baby's 'chest and abdomen' is requested. Figure 4.22: (a) a coin is just visible at the top edge of the film; (b) an extra lateral view showing the coin in the pharynx.

- Other common lodgement sites in the oesophagus are at the bifurcation of the bronchus and the gastro-oesophageal junction.

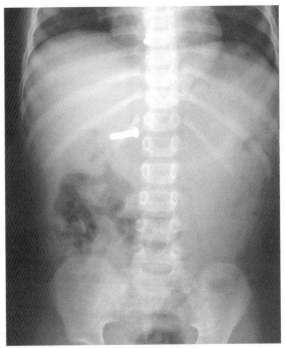

**Figure 4.20**

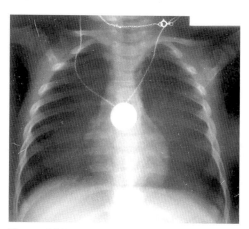

Figure 4.21a

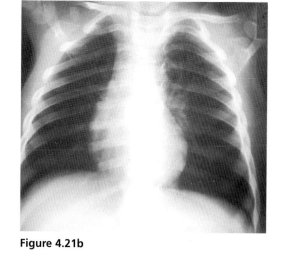

Figure 4.21b

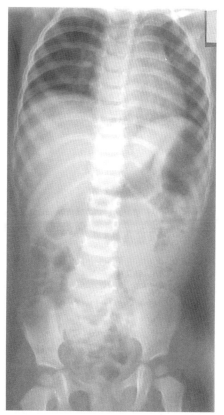

Figure 4.22a

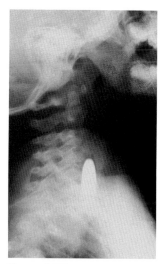

Figure 4.22b

# 5 Neonates

**Introduction**

- The word 'neonate' applies to the first four weeks of life.

- The size of a neonate varies greatly (Fig. 5.1a, b). Positioning is demonstrated on a full-term infant. Almost all x-ray requests are for pre-term infants, which are very tiny and fragile by comparison. (Fig. 5.1c).

- Birth weight can be from less than 1 kg to a possible 4 kg.

- X-raying neonates is the most skilled task required of a radiographer. In no other age group does correct diagnosis and treatment depend so much on high-quality films (Meerstadt & Gyll, 1994).

- Handling of pre-term infants can cause a steep drop in blood oxygen saturation levels. Over-handling can cause cardiorespiratory complications or cerebral haemorrhage.

- Neonates lose heat rapidly. Incubator portholes or flap must not be kept open any longer than is essential for positioning. Incubator heat 30–33°C (85–90°F) can drop 10 degrees in four minutes. Cassettes should be warmed and covered.

- Comfort is important: the infant will not lie still if uncomfortable. Cassette edges should be padded (with gamgee or a nappy). Cotton wool is better than paper towels between the infant and cassette. (See also 'Discussion' on p. 68)

- A full-term infant lifted by a nurse (Fig. 5.2a) or on an incubator sheet by a nurse and radiographer (Fig. 5.2b) for insertion of the cassette.

- A tiny pre-term infant is better not lifted: the cassette is placed under the incubator tray if it is translucent. (See also 'Discussion' on p. 68.)

- The infant's arms and legs should not be extended and held by the nurse as this immobilizes only the limbs, not the body (Fig. 5.3). It is also likely to upset the infant and cause crying/squirming. For the same reason, the pre-term infant's arms should not be held against each side of the head.

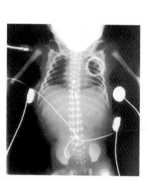
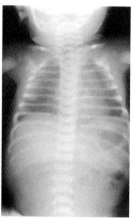
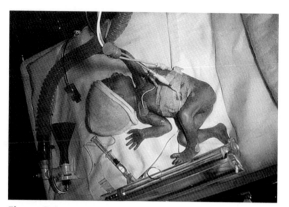

Figure 5.1a

Figure 5.1b

Figure 5.1c

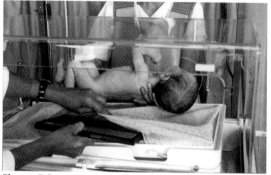

Figure 5.2a

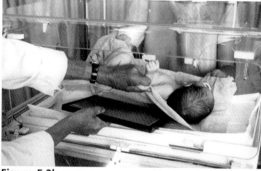

Figure 5.2b

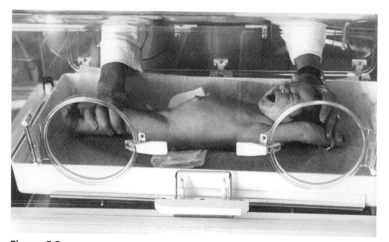

Figure 5.3

**Technical points**

■ The procedure should be standardized: same film/screen combination FFD also milliamps (mA) if possible; kilovoltage (kV) is the only variant.

■ Exposure factors should be noted on the film and used or amended first, if necessary, for all follow-up films.

■ The time the infant is x-rayed should be noted on the film.

■ Care must be taken when digital shuttering is used to ensure that the infant is not irradiated unnecessarily (see Chapter 2, page 28).

■ Hygiene is important: hands must be washed and the cassette wiped with disinfectant. Gonad/thyroid shielding is placed on top of the incubator rather than inside it.

■ The proportions of the chest/abdomen are often misjudged for collimation – approximately one-third to two-thirds (Fig. 5.4a).

■ The x-ray field edges should be seen on the film (Fig. 5.4b). The use of digital shuttering instead of accurate manual collimation ignores the increased radiation dose (Fig. 5.4c).

■ Leads, catheters, etc., must be cleared from the area being x-rayed as much as possible.

*NOTE* There is no need for other staff or parents to leave the room while the infant is x-rayed: the range of scattered radiation is negligible.

**Discussion**

It is worth going to some trouble to identify a form of padding that an infant can lie on rather than a hard cassette and thin paper towel:

■ Some units have very small beanbags that are radiotranslucent.

■ A very thin foam sheet is ideal but must be kept for the use of only one infant at a time.

■ A mattress and incubator tray in an empty incubator can be x-rayed to determine the radiotranslucency and the possibility of artefacts on the film.

■ Mattress covers, folded sheets, etc., can also be tested in the same way.

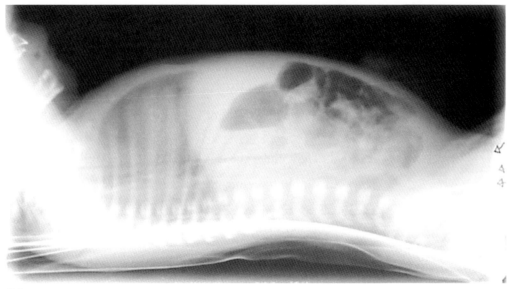

Figure 5.4a

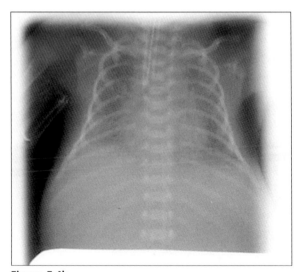

Figure 5.4b

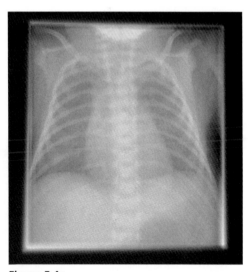

Figure 5.4c

■ A discussion with nursing staff may help to solve this problem.

**Chest**     Reasons for an x-ray request are respiratory distress (there are many causes of this) and congenital heart disease.

***Positioning***     ■ It is essential that the infant lies straight.

■ The head is held (Fig. 5.5a) or propped (Fig. 5.5b) in the AP skull position.

■ A rolled nappy under the legs keeps the pelvis level.

■ The arms should lie symmetrically, slightly away from the sides.

■ The incubator tray is tilted 5–15 degrees (Fig. 5.5a) or the cassette is tilted (Fig. 5.6a), giving the correct AP view (Fig. 5.6b).

■ A very small pre-term infant, especially on a ventilator, needs a cotton wool roll under the neck/shoulders to extend the neck and clear the chin/soft tissues from overlying the lung apices.

■ Ventilator tubing, moved by the nurse, is to be held above the infant's face not left over the upper chest (Fig. 5.7). This may not be possible if high-frequency oscillation ventilation is being used, as the infant's head and neck have to remain in position.

■ If the infant is nursed prone, ask the nurse if it is possible to turn the infant supine. If not, the shoulder at the back of the infant's head should be raised a little to level the chest, and propped in position with a cotton wool or gamgee wedge (Fig. 5.8).

■ The measured dose to the adult's hand is less than 0.002 mSv.

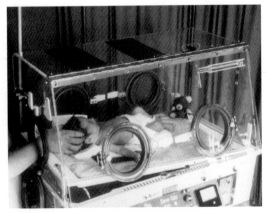

**Figure 5.5a**

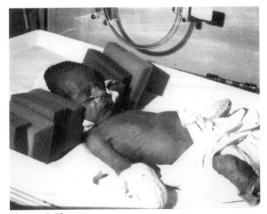

**Figure 5.5b**

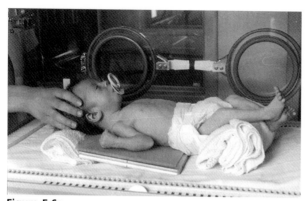

Figure 5.6a

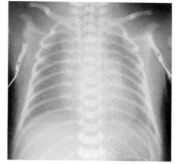

Figure 5.6b

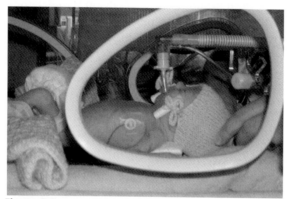

Figure 5.7

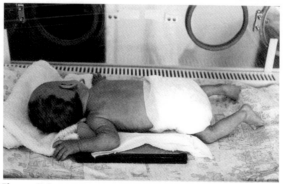

Figure 5.8

***Views and positioning for specific requests***

■ The measured dose to the adult's hand is less than 0.002 mSv.

■ If a request is **to localize an endotracheal tube (ETT)**:
  ● The head should be left lying laterally, i.e. the position in which the infant will be ventilated.
  ● Turning the head straight alters the position of the ETT tip.
  ● The radiograph must be shown immediately to the requesting clinician, in case slight withdrawal is required.

■ Figure 5.9a shows the ETT inserted too far into the right main bronchus causing right upper lobe and left lung collapse. In Fig. 5.9b, the tube has been withdrawn slightly, allowing the lungs to re-expand.

■ A **pneumothorax**, if large, may be seen on a standard AP supine view (Fig. 5.10a); small pneumothoraces may not.
  ● If in doubt, horizontal beam (cross-table) views are taken. Figure 5.10b shows the positioning for Fig. 5.10c radiograph, showing a right lateral pneumothorax.

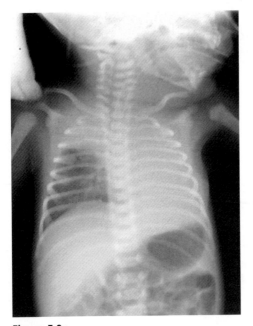

**Figure 5.9a**

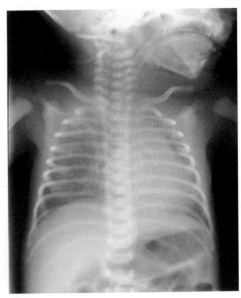

**Figure 5.9b**

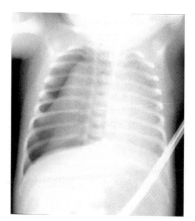

Figure 5.10a

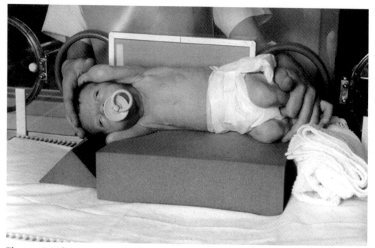

Figure 5.10b

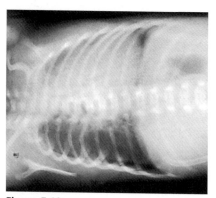

Figure 5.10c

- Note that skin folds can be mistaken for pneumothoraces as there is no subcutaneous fat on a neonate.

■ If an anterior pneumothorax is suspected, a lateral view is taken with a horizontal beam (Fig. 5.11a and b).

■ Exposure factors are **decreased for a lateral view, not increased,** so that the anterior chest wall is seen. This common mistake is shown in Fig.11.6.

*NOTE* In both positions the infant's limbs are not extended. The measure dose to the adult's hands is less than 0.002 mSv.

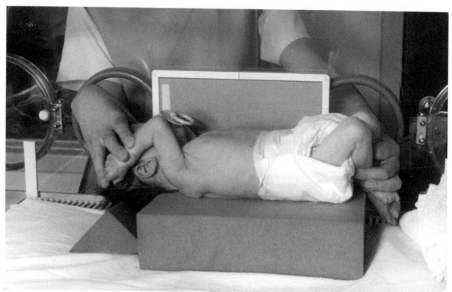

Figure 5.11a

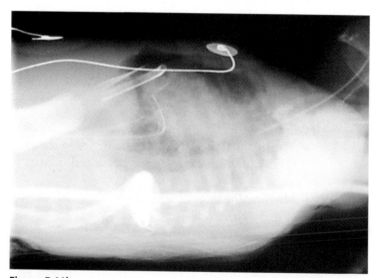

Figure 5.11b

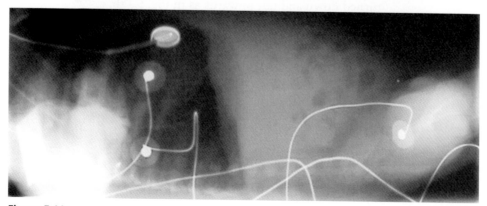

Figure 5.11c

**Common faults**    **Rotation**

■ alters heart size and shape (Fig. 5.12a)

■ distorts the mediastinum, especially the thymus

■ gives differences in translucency between the lungs (Fig. 5.12b); even a very slight degree distorts (Fig. 5.12c).

*Causes*
◆ The head turned to one side.
◆ The hips/shoulders not level.

*Criteria*
◆ The anterior rib ends should be equal in length.
◆ It is often difficult to judge the symmetry of the medial clavicle ends so this is not as accurate a method.

*Correction*
◆ The head held or propped facing forward.
◆ A rolled nappy placed under the legs (Fig. 5.5).

**Lordotic projection**

■ alters heart shape

■ the lower lobes of the lungs are masked by the diaphragm.

*Causes*
◆ The infant and cassette at right angles to the vertical x-ray beam (Fig. 5.13a). Imagine vertical beam and cassette in place for AP view.
◆ Holding the infant's arms above the head, causing the back to arch (Fig. 5.13b).
◆ Centring too low, x-raying the chest with an oblique x-ray beam.

*Criterion*
Posterior ribs should not appear straight; anterior rib ends should be turned down and not upwards as in Fig. 5.13b, c.

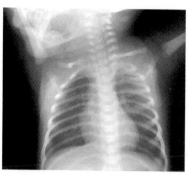

Figure 5.12a

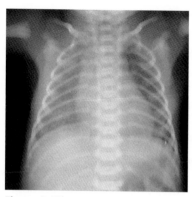

Figure 5.12b

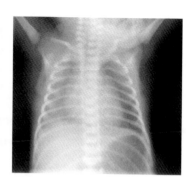

Figure 5.12c

VERTICAL BEAM

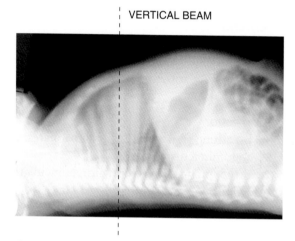

Figure 5.13a

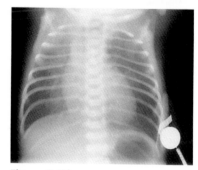

Figure 5.13b

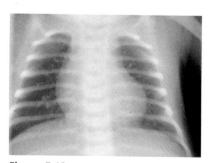

Figure 5.13c

*Correction*
- ◆ Incubator tray tilt of 5–10° head up, or
- ◆ X-ray beam angled 5–10° down, or
- ◆ Cassette tilted, with folded nappy, 5–10° head up.
- ◆ If prone (PA view), the x-ray beam should be angled as for the supine position.

## Exposing on expiration

- ■ Alters the heart shape.

- ■ Obscures lung detail (Fig. 5.14a); repeat on inspiration (Fig. 5.14b).

*Cause*
Mistiming the exposure.

*Criteria*
- ◆ At least eight ribs, and preferably nine, should be seen above the diaphragm. In Fig 5.15 only seven are seen.
- ◆ Some authorities count five anterior rib ends visible as full inspiration.

*Correction*
- ◆ Breathing is diaphragmatic in neonates: expose on maximum abdominal distension.
- ◆ If the infant is on a ventilator, coincide the exposure with needle swing to inspiration.
- ◆ In severe respiratory distress, expose at maximum chest retraction.

**Exposure should not be made if the infant is crying.** Full inspiration when crying overextends the lungs and can suggest pathology. (Ten posterior ribs visible on film.)

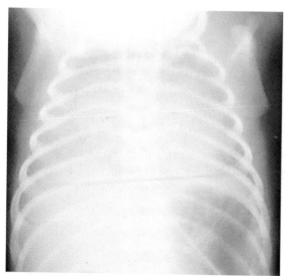

Figure 5.14a

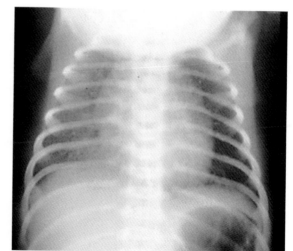

Figure 5.14b

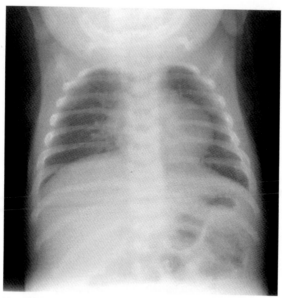

Figure 5.15

### Artefacts

■ Incubator hole (off-centred in all modern incubators):
- over the lower right lung: obvious (Fig. 5.16a)
- over the mediastinum: confusing (Fig. 5.16b)
- over the lower right lung, with a similar round translucency above which is pathological (Fig. 5.16c).

■ Apnoeic mattress: semi-opaque (Figs 5.17, 5.18).

■ Bend in Perspex incubator roof (Fig. 5.19). In Fig. 5.19b the incubator tray is pulled halfway out and the baby x-rayed under the Perspex incubator side.

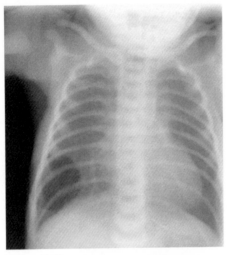

Figure 5.16a

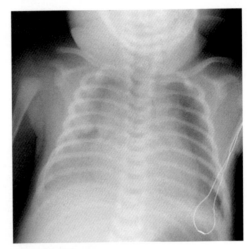

Figure 5.16b

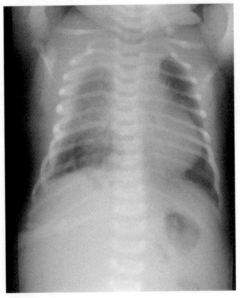

Figure 5.16c

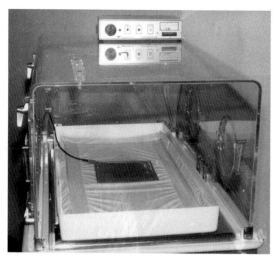

Figure 5.17

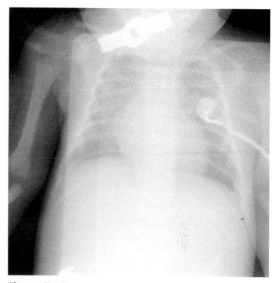

Figure 5.18

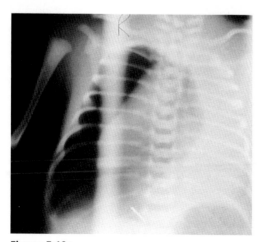

Figure 5.19a

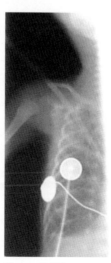
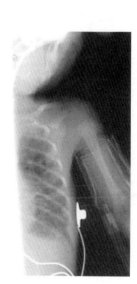

Figure 5.19b

■ Ventilator tubing over lungs (Fig. 5.20a). Tubing disconnected to avoid this but connector still over the lungs (Fig. 5.20b).

■ Cassette nameplate over the lungs (Fig. 5.21).

■ All leads, etc., in Fig. 5.22 – except for ETT and nasojejunal tubes (NJT) – are outside the infant and should have been cleared.

■ The arms can appear as artefacts (Fig. 5.23) and mimic a pneumothorax.

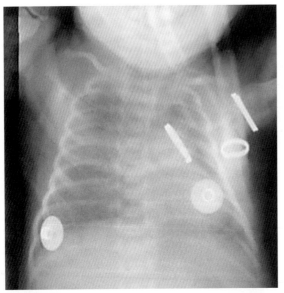

**Figure 5.20a**

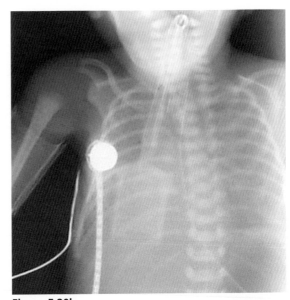

**Figure 5.20b**

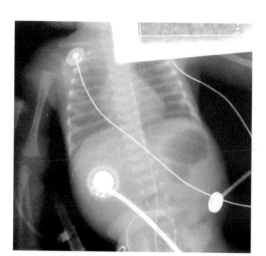

Figure 5.21

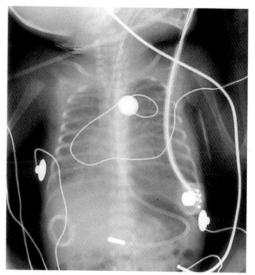

Figure 5.22

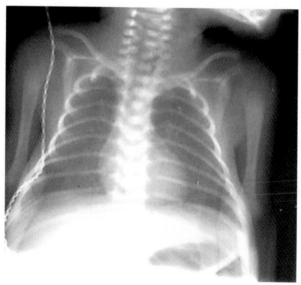

Figure 5.23

## Chest and abdomen on one film

This is needed for two main reasons, which mostly apply to pre-term infants:

- To localize enteral catheters/tubes:
  - umbilical artery catheter (UAC) or umbilical vein catheter (UVC) for taking blood samples
  - NJT for feeding infants with respiratory distress: avoids the risk of regurgitation/inhalation.

- Congenital abnormality involving both the chest and abdomen: oesophageal atresia (OA); tracheo-oesophageal fistula (TOF); and diaphragmatic hernia (DH).

### Technical points

- Centre over the heart (Fig. 5.24). Note the ventilator tubing over the head (not the chest) and ECG leads disconnected to ensure that the x-ray field is clear of artefacts: 800 g infant. The head should be shielded with lead rubber on the incubator top.

- Include the lower abdomen to confirm that the UAC is in the artery not the vein, by showing the pelvic U-bend of the artery. (The tip should be at L3–4 or T6–10, avoiding the renal arteries.)

- Female gonad shielding may obscure the U-bend but male gonads can be excluded by beam collimation.

- Include the chest even if only the abdomen is requested. The tip of the UAC is not visualized in Fig. 5.25a. The UAC is shown too high in the chest in Fig. 5.25b.

- Correct position of NJT (Fig. 5.26). Also present: NGT; ETT; and chest drain. NGT length **outside** infant is left lying underneath left chest: this should have been cleared. Note that both male and female gonads can be excluded by beam collimation.

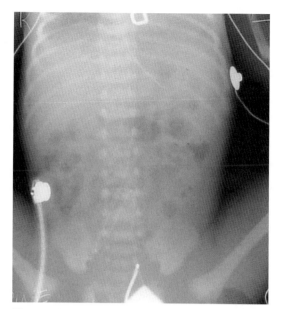

Figure 5.25a

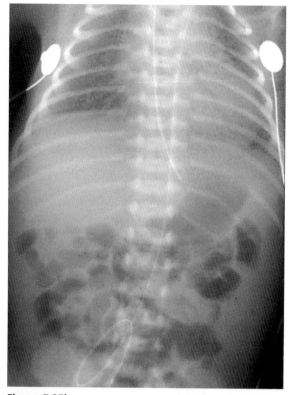

Figure 5.25b

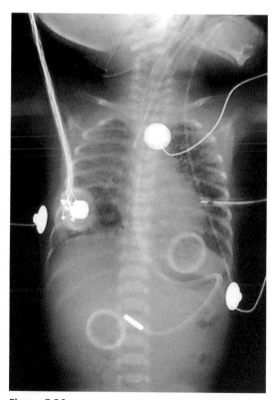

Figure 5.26

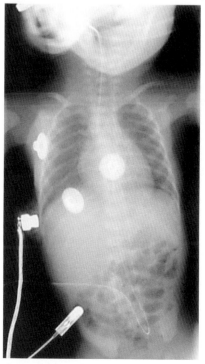

Figure 5.24

**Oesophageal atresia and tracheo-oesophageal fistula**

■ OA: blind upper and lower ends to the oesophagus.

■ OA + TOF: fistula to trachea from either or both blind end(s).

■ TOF: fistula to trachea from patent oesophagus (very rare).

■ An opaque catheter is passed into the blind upper pouch and the infant is x-rayed.

**Technical points**

■ It is essential that facial soft tissues and the mandible do not overlie and mask the tube in the upper pouch (Meerstadt & Gyll, 1994).

■ Include the upper abdomen to show if there is gas in the stomach: this indicates a fistula from the trachea to the lower oesophageal pouch (Fig. 5.27), the commonest (at 80–90%) of five variations.

■ Collimate beam to exclude the gonads. Note how distorted the chest appears from inadequate positioning (Fig. 5.27).

**Diaphragmatic hernia**

■ Congenital non-closure of foramen in the diaphragm, causing intrusion of the abdominal organs into the chest.

■ Degree of herniation varies. A large hernia may contain part of the small or large gut, stomach and spleen, filling the entire hemithorax (Fig. 5.28): a life-threatening surgical emergency.

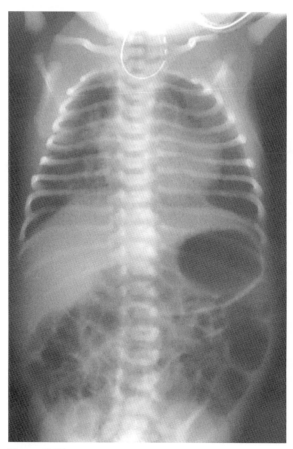

Figure 5.27

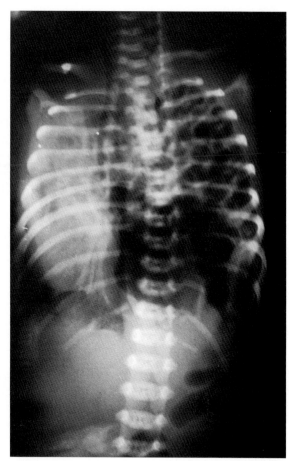

Figure 5.28

***Common faults***

■ Using the same exposure for the chest and abdomen of a full-term infant 'blacks out' the lung detail (Fig. 5.29). This is acceptable only if the request is just for localization of tubes/catheters.

■ Centring below the diaphragm and/or raising the infant's arms will cause a lordotic projection (Fig. 5.29).

■ The head has been irradiated unnecessarily (Fig. 5.30). There is no lead rubber on the incubator top. NOTE: Films like this are not seen when digital radiography is used. The image is accurately collimated by shuttering post-processing. The possibility still exists of the infant being over-irradiated. This should not be overlooked (see Chapter 2).

■ Equipment leads have not been cleared (Fig. 5.31). NGT and ETT are the only tubes **inside** the infant; all others are **outside**.

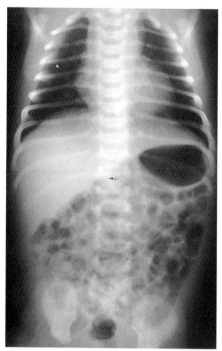

Figure 5.29

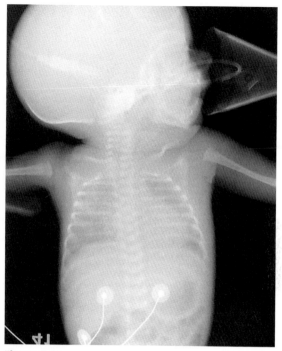

Figure 5.30

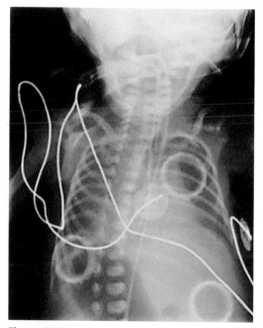

Figure 5.31

**Abdomen**

Reasons for x-ray requests:

- Distended abdomen:
  - intestinal obstruction
  - abdominal mass.

- Necrotizing enterocolitis (NEC): this may cause perforation of the bowel.

**Positioning**

- The infant must lie straight for the AP view (Fig. 5.32). A lateral view with vertical beam is very rarely needed (Fig. 5.33a). Note how low the rectum is: collimation is not to the lower edge of the abdomen bulge (Fig. 5.33b).

- The infant's elbows/knees are left flexed. The hips are extended, clear of abdomen for both views.

- Note the holder's finger between infant's ankles/wrists: it is then easier to keep the arms and legs symmetrical.

- The measured dose to the adult's hands is 0.003 mSv (Figs 5.32, 5.33).

- The cassette edges need to be padded with a nappy or gamgee.

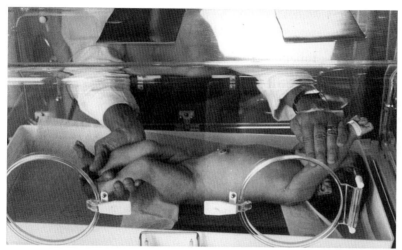

Figure 5.32a

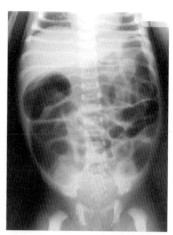

Figure 5.32b

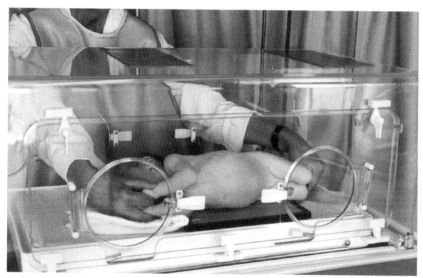

Figure 5.33a

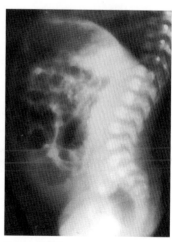

Figure 5.33b

*Common faults*

■ Too small an x-ray field, excluding the rectum (Fig. 5.34a) or diaphragm (Fig 5.34b).

■ Too large an x-ray field, including the chest (Fig. 5.35).

■ Too tight, lateral collimation (Fig. 5.36). (See Fig. 5.4, page 69, for chest/abdomen proportions).

■ Misplaced gonad protection (Fig. 5.37). It may be essential to demonstrate the presence of gas in the rectum.

■ Name over the rectum (Fig. 5.38). The cassette has been reversed with the namespace at the bottom, as for adults.

*Artefacts*

■ tubes/catheters/leads (Fig. 5.39)

■ clip marker (Fig. 5.40)

■ tape measure (Fig. 5.41)

■ namespace and lead letters (Fig. 5.42).

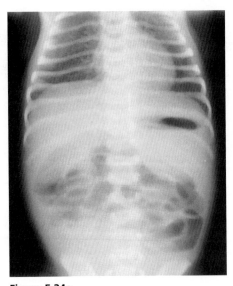

**Figure 5.34a**

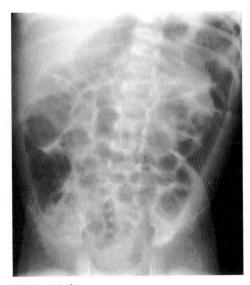

**Figure 5.34b**

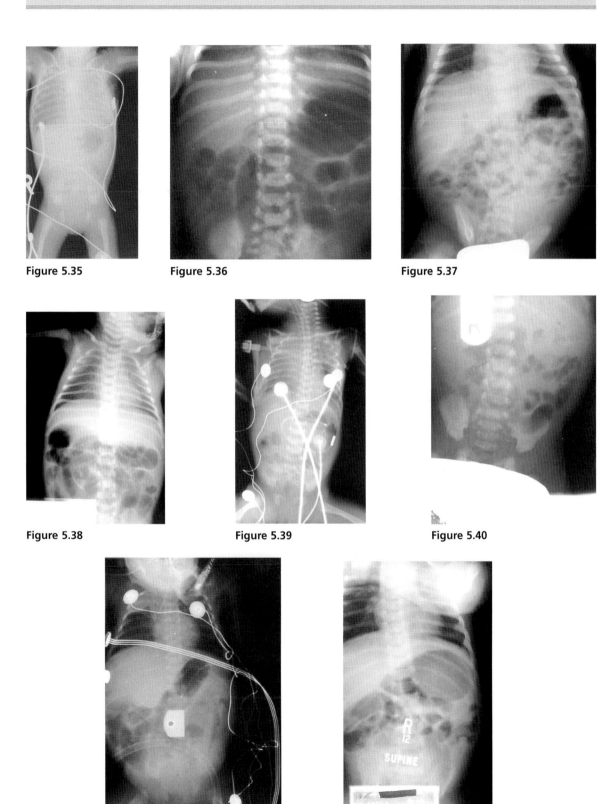

Figure 5.35

Figure 5.36

Figure 5.37

Figure 5.38

Figure 5.39

Figure 5.40

Figure 5.41

Figure 5.42

***Views and positioning for specific requests***

Decubitus horizontal beam (cross-table) views have replaced traditional erect views (even on full-term babies) for fluid levels or pneumoperitoneum because:

■ far less handling is needed

■ there is no heat loss with the infant positioned in the incubator

■ accurate positioning is much easier so a better film is achieved.

### Positioning for horizontal beam AP view

■ Elbows/knees flexed, hips extended clear of the abdomen (Fig. 5.43).

■ The infant's back must be flat against the cassette (Fig. 5.43).

■ If in a closed incubator, the infant must be raised above the level of the porthole fastening clips on a foam pad or folded nappies (Fig. 5.43).

■ It is essential to collimate within the cassette edges (as always).

■ Fluid level in gut obstruction (Fig. 5.44a).

■ 'Tell-tale triangle' sign in perforation (Fig. 5.44b).

■ Duodenal atresia 'double bubble' sign (Fig. 5.44c).

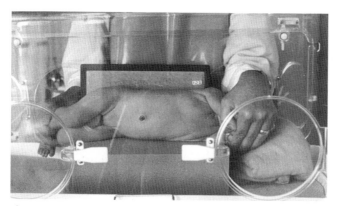

Figure 5.43

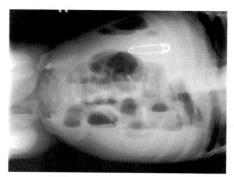

Figure 5.44a

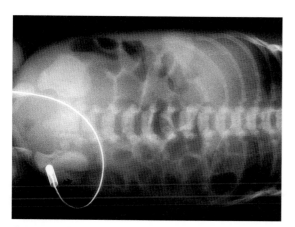

Figure 5.44b

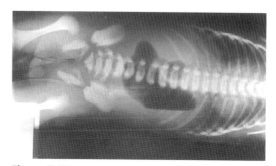

Figure 5.44c

**Common faults**

- ■ *NOTE* The term 'lateral decubitus' is frequently misused. It does not mean 'lateral view'. It means an AP view with the infant lying on one side (which side must be identified). A horizontal beam lateral view is taken in the dorsal decubitus position (lying on the back). The letters HBL have been seen written by radiographers on AP views.

- ■ Hips not extended so the legs obscure the lower abdomen (Fig. 5.45).

- ■ The infant's back is not wholly against the cassette: pelvis rotated forward. Therefore not a standard AP view (Fig. 5.46).

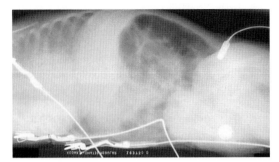

Figure 5.45

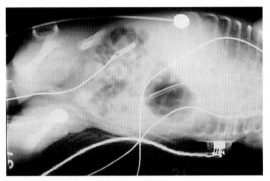

Figure 5.46

***Positioning for horizontal beam lateral view***

- Elbows/knees are flexed and hips semi-extended (Fig. 5.47a).

- The infant must be raised above the level of the porthole fastening clips (Fig. 5.47a).

- Pneumoperitoneum in bowel perforation is better seen in this than in an AP view (Fig. 5.47b, c).

- Advantage: less handling than for an AP view.

### Common faults

- Exposure factors must be **decreased** from AP, not increased as with adults (Fig. 5.48a). It is essential to be able to see the anterior abdominal wall (Fig. 5.48b). The spine should be barely visible. Figure 5.48 shows an increase of 8 kV for the exposure.

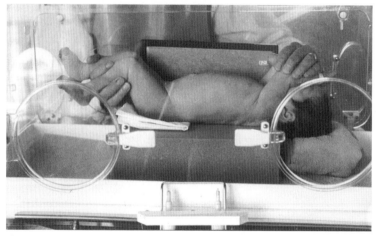

**Figure 5.47a**

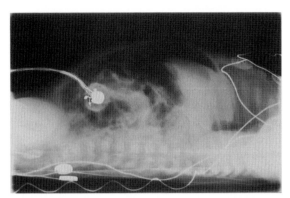

Figure 5.47b

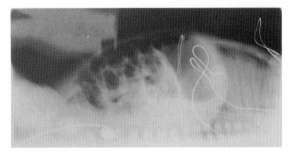

Figure 5.47c

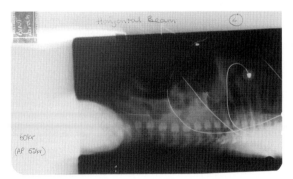

Figure 5.48a

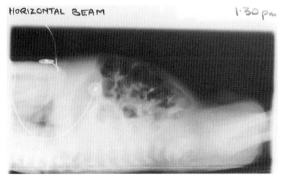

Figure 5.48b

*Artefacts*

These are the same as for the AP view with vertical beam (ECG leads, etc.; Fig. 5.49), plus mattress and incubator tray edges (Fig. 5.50a) and the porthole rim and clip (Fig. 5.50b).

*Anorectal anomalies (imperforate anus)*

There are many variants. The main division is into a high or low category, i.e. the gut ends above or below the pelvic floor. The high type needs abdominal surgery.

- Diagnosis is usually made by sonography. The radiographic technique is described for occasions when this is not available.

- The infant must be at least 18 hours old, preferably 24, for swallowed air to reach the rectum.

- The infant must be positioned and left inverted for 2–10 minutes before a horizontal beam lateral view can be taken.

- The prone position, over a 45° pad in the incubator is now the **accepted standard positioning** (Fig. 5.51). There is less handling, no heat loss and less upset for the infant. (The traditional position was with the infant held upside-down by the legs with an opaque marker on the anus.)

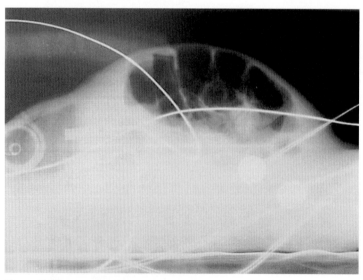

**Figure 5.49**

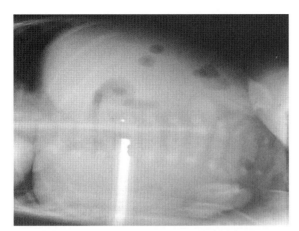

Figure 5.50a

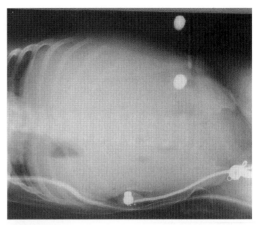

Figure 5.50b

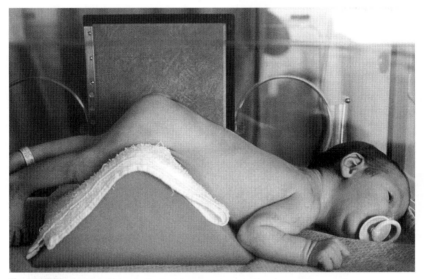

Figure 5.51a

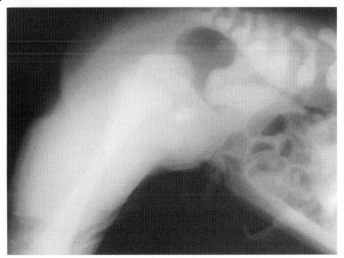

Figure 5.51b

# 6 The skull

**Introduction**

- The commonest reason for an x-ray request is 'head injury'.

- The routine x-raying of children with minor head injury is no longer acceptable practice (WHO, 1987).

- The presence of a fracture in the adult skull indicates high risk of brain damage but **the opposite is true in children** (DeLacey *et al.*, 1980).

- A fracture is important only if it is depressed or if NAI is suspected.

- CT is the imaging method of choice for severe injuries.

*Positioning*

- Infants under 3 months old are best x-rayed after a feed as they will then sleep through the examination if wrapped up and comfortable (Fig. 6.1). No restraint is needed. A baby-sized skull foam pad is used for the AP position.

- A 15° foam pad is used for the lateral view with the infant lying on one side (Fig. 6.2).

- Aged 3 months and over, wrapping up is not advisable as this will probably cause crying and/or struggling.

- Immobilization of a 3-month-old baby in the correct position is achieved with a bottle (Fig. 6.3): sandbags over the legs, skull foam pad for the AP position, 35° foam pad under the shoulder for the lateral position: arms are not restrained.

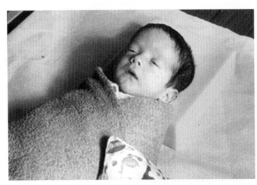

**Figure 6.1a**

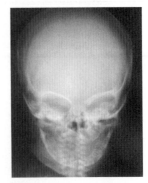

**Figure 6.1b**

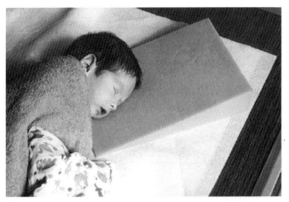

Figure 6.2a

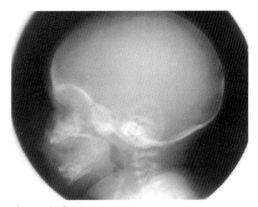

Figure 6.2b

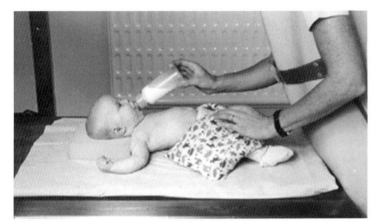

Figure 6.3a

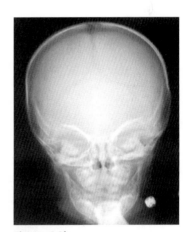

Figure 6.3b

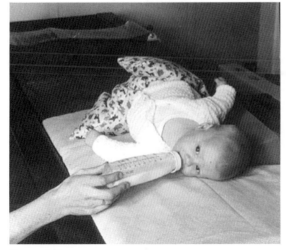

Figure 6.3c

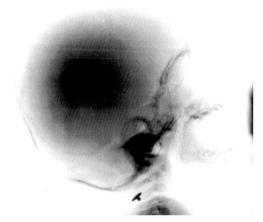

Figure 6.3d

■ It is impossible to hold a struggling baby or toddler in position by force. **Avoidance of upset** and a very short exposure time are of the utmost importance. Figure 6.4 is a lateral view of a 6-month-old baby.

■ Positioning for an older baby (aged 9 months) is shown in Fig. 6.5. A foam pad under the Bucky band immobilizes the lower half of the body, the mother keeps in eye contact and the head is held AP with foam pads. The child's attention is caught and held by a toy at the table's edge for the lateral view. 45° foam pad under the opposite shoulder. Note: the dummy/pacifier and that the infant's arms are not restrained.

■ Positioning of a 2-year-old (Fig. 6.6a). The mother is at the end of the table (not in the centre) so that she can stand in line with the child's head to see that it is not rotated for an AP view.

■ Bucky band and foam pads are used as before; the head is on a ring foam pad. Note the placing of the foam pads so that the child's view is not restricted nor her ears covered (see also Fig. 6.5a). Figure 6.6b shows the mother at the tableside for lateral view, the 45° foam pad under the child's opposite shoulder and adult's finger on the jaw to prevent the head turning.

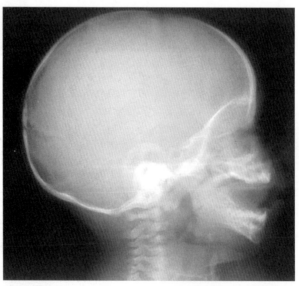

**Figure 6.4**

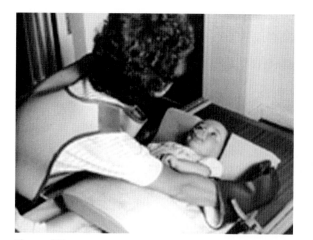

Figure 6.5a

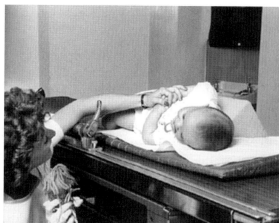

Figure 6.5b

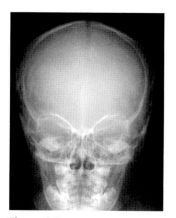

Figure 6.5c

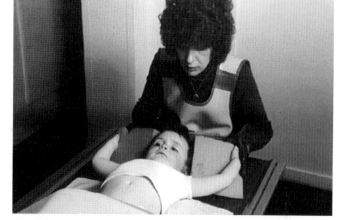

Figure 6.6a

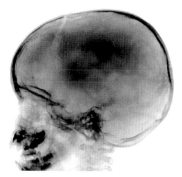

Figure 6.5d

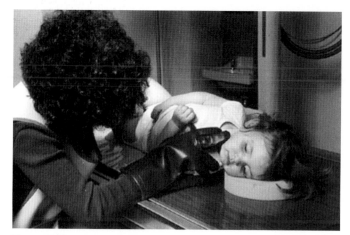

Figure 6.6b

- A 4-year-old in position (Fig. 6.7). The head is on a skull or ring foam pad; the 45° foam pad under the far shoulder for the lateral view.

- An AP view is recommended, rather than PA, for under 5 or 6 years of age. The increase in radiation to the lens of the eyes is negligible by comparison with the threshold dose for cataract production: about 1 mSv as compared with 5500 mSv (ICRP, 1969).

- A child over 6 years old is x-rayed as an adult.

- Standard routine views are AP or PA and lateral. Semi-axial (Towne's view) is supplementary (WHO,1987).

- Use of a skull unit is inadvisable for children younger than 6 years old. Horizontal beam lateral, as for adults, is unnecessary, as sphenoids are not aerated until after 6 years of age.

- The head is fully grown by approximately 6 years of age, therefore adult exposure factors are needed. Figure 6.8 is of a 5-year-old.

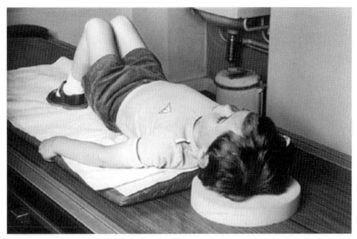

Figure 6.7a

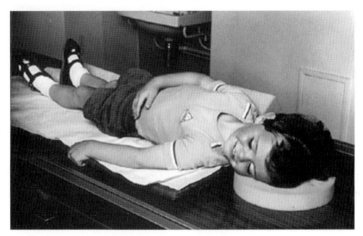

Figure 6.7b

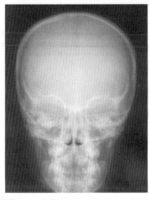

Figure 6.8a

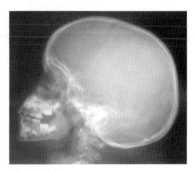

Figure 6.8b

**Common faults**

- rotated (Fig. 6.9)

- too large a field, also rotated (Fig. 6.10)

- adult's hands irradiated (Fig. 6.11)

- zip, poppers, etc., over Towne's view:
  - zip top in the foramen magnum because the tube was angled (Fig. 6.12a)
  - collection of jewellery (Fig. 6.13).

- hair braids (Fig. 6.14).

**Facial bones and the jaw**

Injuries to the face and jaw are much less common in children; x-ray examination as for adults. Nasal bones, even if fractured, are not x-rayed (Raby *et al.*, 1995).

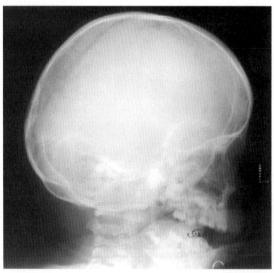

**Figure 6.9**

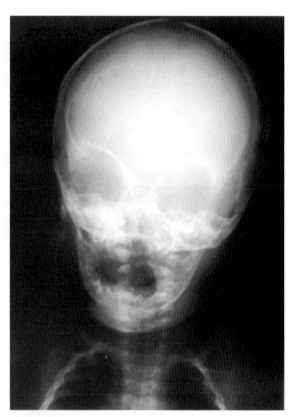

**Figure 6.10**

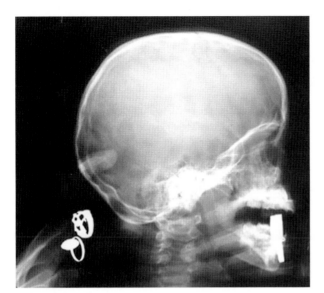

Figure 6.11

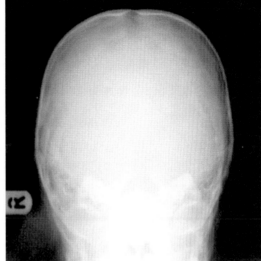

Figure 6.12

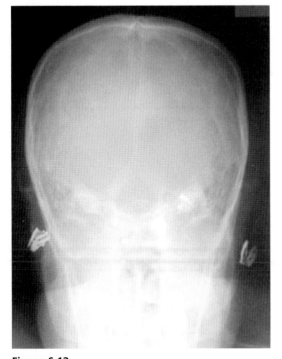

Figure 6.13

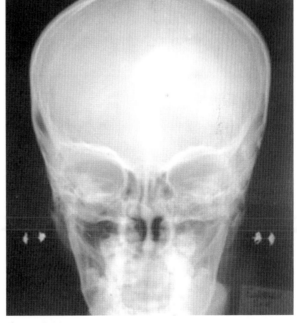

Figure 6.14

## OTOLARYNGOLOGY

**Sinuses**

- Are usually x-rayed only if requested by an ENT consultant.

- One view (occipitomental) is taken erect (Fig. 6.15).

- Should not be x-rayed in under 5-year olds (Royal College of Radiologists, 1998). Sinuses are poorly developed and mucosal thickening can be normal.

- Positioning: base line angulation is 10° less than for adults (Fig. 6.16). Compare the position of the child's chin in (a) over-tilted and (b) correct positioning.

- Figure 6.15b is of a 10-year-old boy. Note normal undeveloped frontal sinuses.

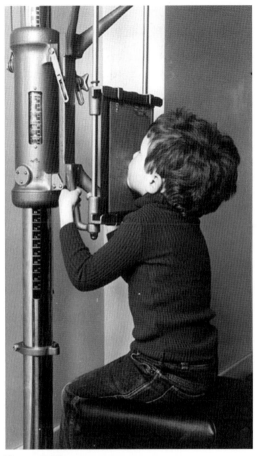

Figure 6.15a

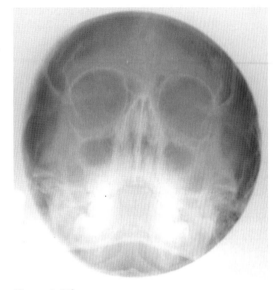

Figure 6.15b

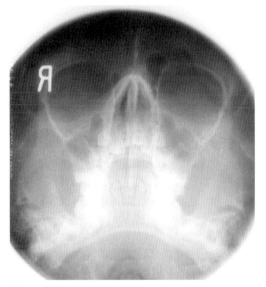

Figure 6.16a

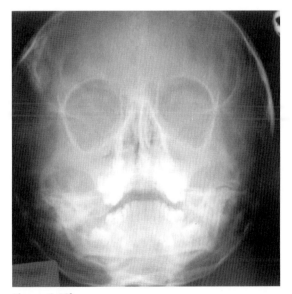

Figure 6.16b

**The postnasal space (PNS)**

- Usually x-rayed only if requested by an ENT consultant (to show enlarged adenoids). Positioning is shown in Fig. 6.17a.

- One lateral view, collimated horizontally to the angle of the mandible so as to exclude the thyroid, and vertically so as to avoid irradiating eyes (Fig. 6.17).

- PNS must be air-filled to demonstrate enlarged adenoids; seen at the centre of the mandibular ramus.

- The child should breathe in through the nose during exposure. If the nose is blocked, the child should breathe in and hold the breath with mouth shut.

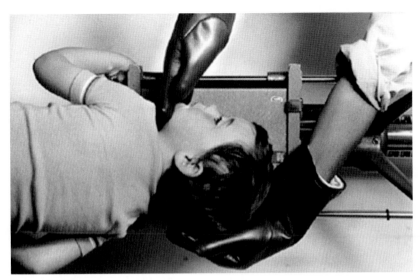

Figure 6.17a

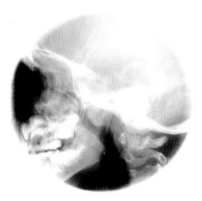

Figure 6.17b

# 7 The spine

**Introduction**
- Injuries are rare, causes:
  - fall from a considerable height
  - Road Traffic Accident (RTA).
- Backache is rare in children without underlying pathology; needs investigation.
- Spinal cord tumours are very rare. Cord pathology is investigated by sonography in infants and by magnetic resonance imaging (MRI) in children.

**Positioning**
- The same as for adults.
- No separate L5–S1 view needed until the teenage years.
- Erect positioning required for some orthopaedic conditions.

**Pathology**
- Infection: radionuclide imaging is preferable to radiography.
- Congenital abnormalities:
  - hemivertebra, causes scoliosis
  - spina bifida: varying degrees of severity.
  - Figure 7.1 shows severe spina bifida with kyphosis.
  - Figure 7.2 shows a postoperative PA view of a 4-day-old infant, prone, in an incubator.

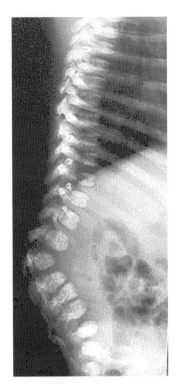 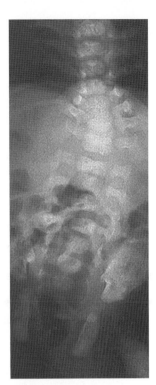

Figure 7.1a                              Figure 7.1b

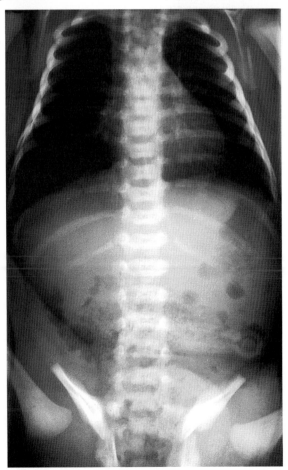

Figure 7.2

- Tethered cord:
  - Arches fuse at 1–2 years. Non-closure cannot be diagnosed radiologically before this, unless gross. Defect visible in a 2-year-old (Fig. 7.3).
  - Spina bifida occulta (Fig. 7.4) no significance.
  - The cord should move from top of third lumbar vertebra to bottom of first by the age of 5 years. In some children there may be abnormal adhesion of the free end of the cord, so it will stretch as the child grows, causing neurological symptoms; investigated by MRI.

*Scoliosis*  **Types: idiopathic, acquired paralytic and congenital**

- The commonest is idiopathic: lateral curvature of the spine with rotation of normal vertebrae (Fig. 7.5).

- Onset at puberty, mostly in girls.

- Occurs in three age groups:
  - infantile: a simple C curve up to 3 years of age; approximately 10% of cases get worse
  - juvenile at about 5–6 years
  - adolescent, presenting at puberty, by far the most frequent age of onset.

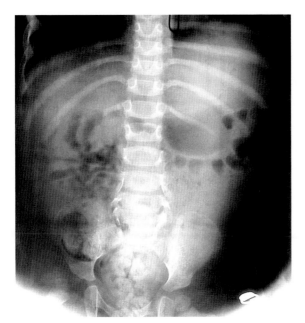

Figure 7.3

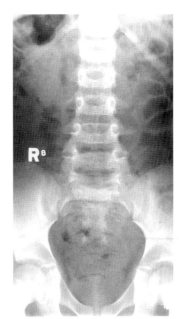

Figure 7.4

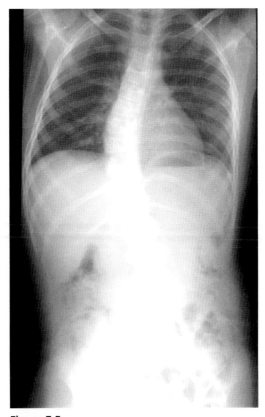

Figure 7.5

### Technical points

First x-ray examination: erect, from level of the seventh cervical vertebra to iliac crests, shoes off and gonads screened (Fig. 7.6):

■ High kV (100+) reduces radiation dose and contrast, so thoracic and lumbar vertebrae are equally visualized.

■ A 2 m (6 ft) air gap is considered better than a grid.

■ AP/PA view controversy: a PA view reduces dose to the developing breasts but increases dose to the spinal cord. Authorities differ in preference.

■ Lateral view for associated kyphosis.

■ Iliac crest apophyses included to check maturity, fusion coincides with the end of spinal growth (Fig. 7.7).

■ Treatment is bracing for the idiopathic type, surgery mainly for the paralytic; Harrington and/or Luque rods (Fig. 7.8).

*NOTE* Lateral-flexion views are taken only at regional scoliosis centres, not for follow-up at local general hospitals.

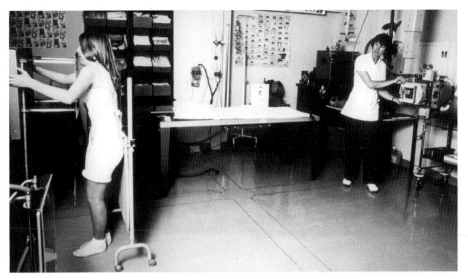

**Figure 7.6**

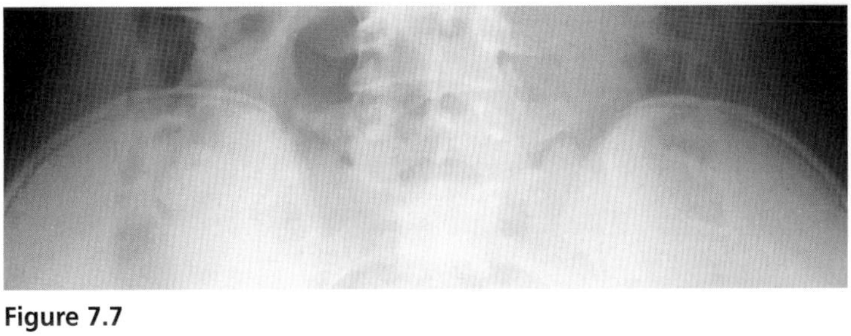

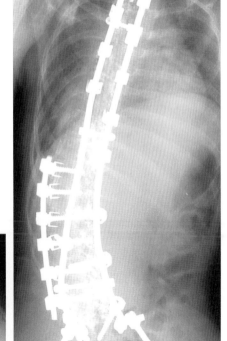

**Figure 7.7**

**Figure 7.8**

- Follow-up imaging: Surface Topography (Quantec®) Imaging; no radiation dose (Fig. 7.9).

- Only a PA or AP view for follow-up; no lateral view if surface topography is not available.

**Other spinal conditions**

- Spondylolisthesis rarely occurs in childhood. The usual views required are lateral (centred on lumbosacral junction) and oblique views of the lumbar vertebrae.

- Trauma is very rare. Figure 7.10 shows fracture of the first lumbar vertebra: (excellent radiographic collimation and gonad protection). Note visibility of L5–S1 with the same exposure factors as for L1–L4.

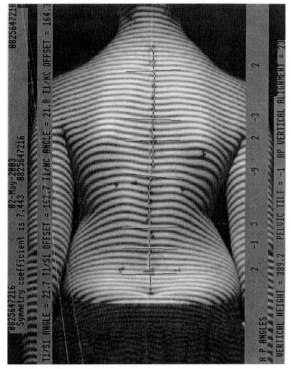

Figure 7.9

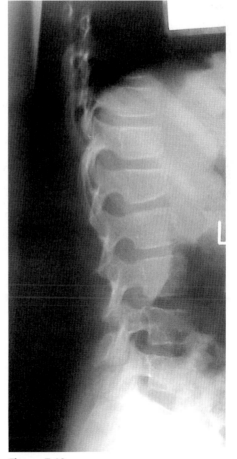

Figure 7.10

## PELVIS

- Radiography of a child's whole pelvis, as opposed to an AP view of hip joints, is seldom required.

- The main reason for x-raying the pelvis is suspected injury caused by an RTA.

- Fracture or dislocation is rare; 80–90% have multiple injuries, especially of the head and viscera (Thornton & Gyll, 1999). These are more important than pelvic fractures. Unlike in adults, fractures are rarely displaced enough to need reduction (Thornton & Gyll, 1999).

- The approximate age range is 6–16 years.

- The most common fracture is of the pubic rami. Care is needed to ensure that the fracture site is not obscured by gonad protection. Figure 7.11 shows a 9-year-old girl who was knocked down by a car.
  - AP view of the pelvis, thought to demonstrate a fractured neck of right femur. Further views were taken.
  - AP and lateral views of the femoral neck, using gonad protection. The girl was transferred to another hospital and put in traction. Because of this transfer, the films were kept in the ward and not reported.
  - Check of the film two weeks later revealed the true injury: fractured pubic rami, which was also evident on the original film of the pelvis but was missed then.

- Positioning is the same as for adults. Only one AP view is taken.

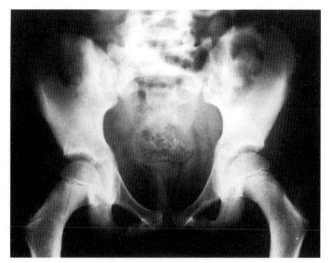

Figure 7.11a

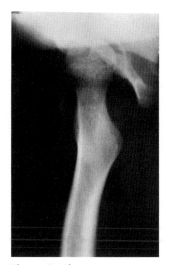

Figure 7.11b

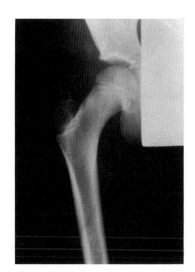

Figure 7.11c

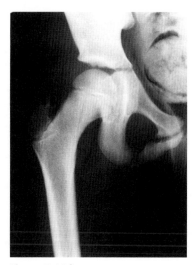

Figure 7.11d

# 8 The arm

**The incidence of all fractures is age related.**

## Shoulder and humerus

Likely fractures include:

- clavicle: all ages
- upper humeral epiphysis: teenage
- upper humeral metaphysis: five years and above
- dislocation: teenage.

Comparison views of the opposite side should not be routinely taken (WHO, 1987; Royal College of Radiologists, 1995).

### Under 15 months of age

- The request is usually for 'whole arm'.
- One anteroposterior (AP) view is enough if a fracture is seen.
- Figure 8.1a shows a 9-month-old baby positioned, attention distracted by a squeaker (which aids immobilization).

NOTE:
- The cassette corner under the baby is padded by a pillow.
- A 35° foam pad under the opposite side to rotate the trunk slightly towards the injured arm.
- A Bucky band, with a foam pad underneath, is tightened across the hips for immobilization.

- If a fracture is present, it is almost always of the clavicle (Fig. 8.1b).
- A fractured humeral shaft is suspicious of non-accidental injury (NAI).

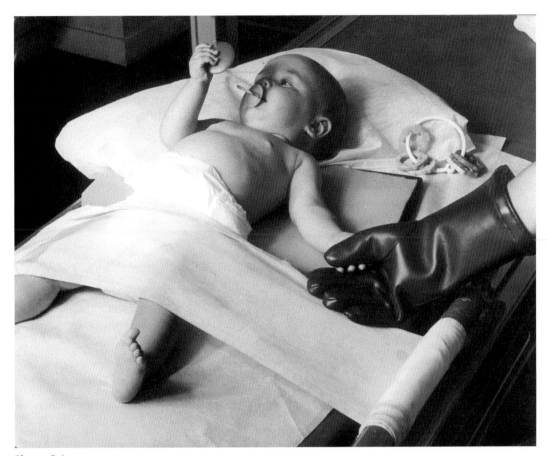

Figure 8.1a

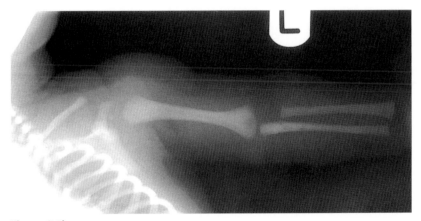

Figure 8.1b

### Common faults

■ The clavicle is obscured by the namespace or the baby's chin (Fig. 8.2).

■ Breathing blur, and x-ray field too large (Fig. 8.3).

■ Rotating a baby's wrist does not give a lateral view of the arm (Fig. 8.4). Also, the clavicle is not seen in this film.

### Danger/cruelty

The baby's arm is rotated for an unnecessary second view (Fig. 8.5). Compare the upper half of humerus in both films: it has hardly moved. **Rotation pivots on the fracture.**

### Radiation protection

■ X-ray field collimated to the arm. Ribs should not be included.

■ The radiation dose is halved by omitting the second standard view if a fracture is seen on the first film. This should be the protocol agreed between radiologists and A & E consultants. It also avoids unnecessary suffering and danger, as seen in Fig. 8.5.

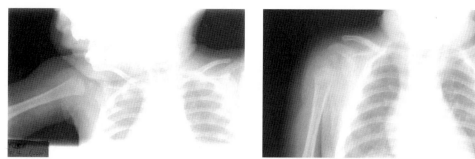

Figure 8.2

Figure 8.3

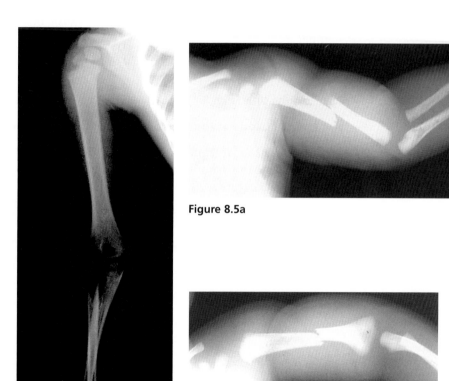

Figure 8.4

Figure 8.5a

Figure 8.5b

*15 months to 3 years*

- The usual history is 'not using arm'.

- Likely injury is fractured clavicle or 'pulled elbow' (see p. 140).

- One AP view erect is possible, even as young as 15 months, if a baby-seat for erect chest radiography is available (Fig. 8.6a). Supine positioning can give a false positive appearance, as with the 3-year-old in Fig. 8.6b.

- Exposure factors and focal film distance are as for chest.

- Collimation should include the clavicle and humerus on the injured side only.

- A baby's attention is attracted by a toy or music box on the x-ray tube.

## Common faults

- Breathing blur (Fig. 8.7).

- Clavicle fracture at the edge of the x-ray field (Fig. 8.8).

- X-ray field too large: midshaft clavicle fracture (Fig. 8.9). X-ray request probably 'shoulder and arm'. Requests must specify suspected injury for correct views to be taken.

## Radiation protection

- The child is over-irradiated if the x-ray field is not collimated accurately.

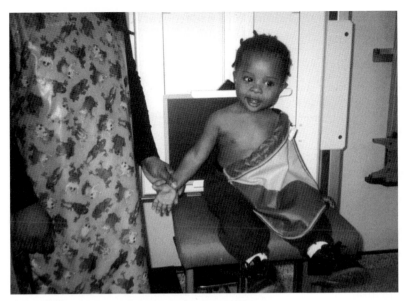

Figure 8.6a

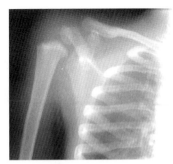

Figure 8.6b

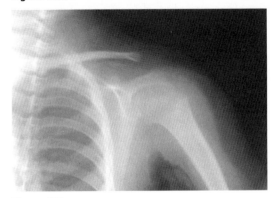

Figure 8.7

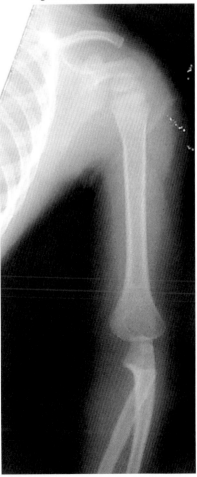

Figure 8.8

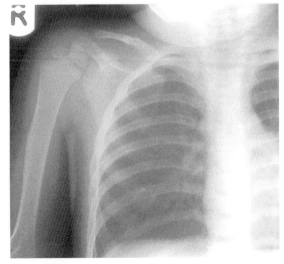

Figure 8.9

A 2-year-old positioned sitting on a padded seat at the chest stand (Fig. 8.10):

■ Usual history is 'not using arm'.

■ The likely injury is a fractured clavicle or 'pulled elbow' (see p. 140).

■ The dose to the adult holder's hands is not more than 0.002 mSv (Gyll & Blake, 1986).

A 3-year-old in position (Fig. 8.11). The x-ray field is collimated diagonally to shoulder or arm:

■ Usual history of fall from a climbing frame, tree, etc.

■ The injury site is often not localized clinically.

■ The most likely injury is fractured clavicle.

■ Note the lead rubber apron: it is difficult to exclude the chest by collimation.

An extra view is required if there is strong clinical suspicion of fracture but the first film is negative:

■ The child is positioned as for the AP view.

■ The x-ray tube is angled 10–12° cephalad (Fig. 8.12).

■ The second view shows a midshaft greenstick fracture (Fig. 8.13).

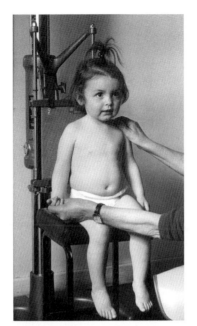

Figure 8.10

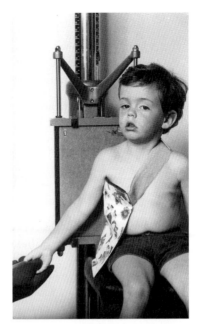

Figure 8.11

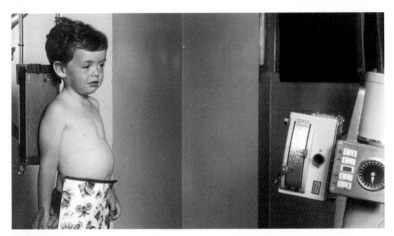

Figure 8.12

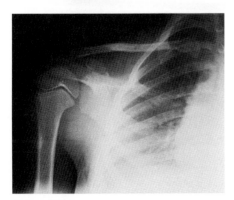

Figure 8.13a

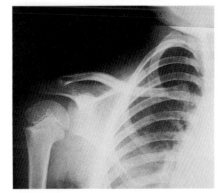

Figure 8.13b

### *Clavicle*    **4 years of age and over**

■ A well-collimated AP view of the clavicle is possible because the injury is localized to the clavicle on the request form. Figure 8.14 shows a radiograph of a 5-year-old boy.

■ An inaccurately centred AP view (Fig. 8.15), probably because the injury is not localized clinically.

■ An AP view of a 12-year-old's shoulder (Fig. 8.16a). Positioning was the same as for an adult with slight rotation to the affected side. The fracture was not demonstrated. The injury was not localized on the request form ('shoulder') so an incorrect view was taken.

■ The film was repeated with the child positioned PA, so that the clavicle is parallel to the cassette: fracture seen (Fig. 8.16b).

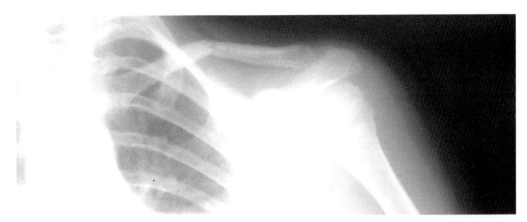

Figure 8.14

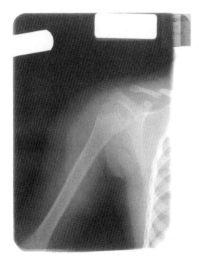

Figure 8.15

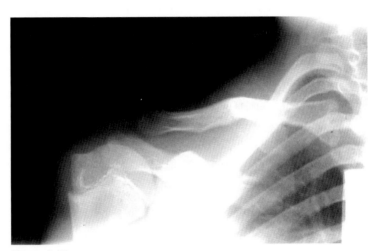

Figure 8.16a

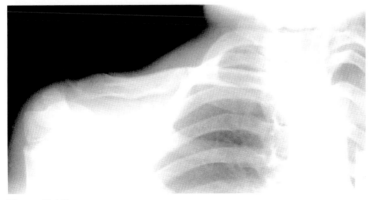

Figure 8.16b

***Older child: 6 years of age and over***

- At this age, injury can be localized. If 'shoulder and humerus' is requested, only the upper half of humerus need be included. If 'elbow and humerus' is requested, include only the lower half.

- If 'shoulder, humerus and elbow' is requested, ask the child where it hurts (Fig. 8.17): the request should have been localized to the shoulder.

- An AP scout view of the whole clavicle and upper humerus is taken if the injury is not localized on the request form (Fig. 8.18).

- If a fractured clavicle or shoulder dislocation is demonstrated, a second view is not needed.

- With a fractured humeral epiphysis or metaphysis, the choice of positioning for a second view depends on whether pain is caused.
  - With a buckle fracture, internal rotation is often painless (Fig. 8.19).
  - For a complete (Fig. 8.20a) or epiphyseal fracture (Fig. 8.20b), the modified lateral scapula view is recommended. (See Fig. 8.21.)

- An axial view (inferosuperior or superoinferior) should not be attempted for any clinically suspected injury to the upper humerus.

*NOTE* Manipulation under anaesthetic is very rarely necessary for epiphyseal or metaphyseal fractures, and never for a buckle fracture. A second view may be considered justified only if requested by an orthopaedic surgeon intending manipulation.

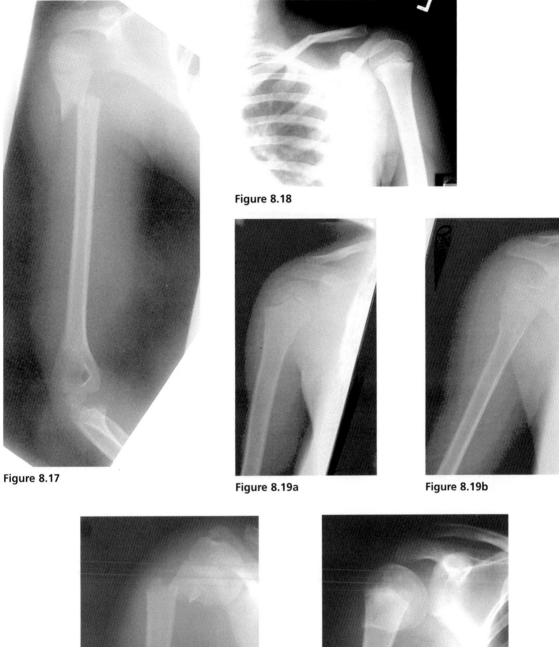

Figure 8.17

Figure 8.18

Figure 8.19a

Figure 8.19b

Figure 8.20a

Figure 8.20b

- For the modified lateral scapula view, the child first supports the forearm with the other hand (Fig. 8.21a). He is then turned to face the cassette and leans towards the injured side to separate arm from body (Fig. 8.21b).

  This gives a true lateral view of the humerus (Fig. 8.22).

- From 9 or 10 years of age, the upper and lower humerus need different exposure factors (Fig. 8.23).

- Appropriate collimation, centring and exposure will give a true lateral view of the upper end of humerus or of the elbow.

- Soft tissue swelling after a fracture needs increased exposure (Fig. 8.24). It can be gross.

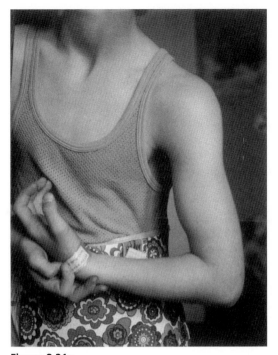

Figure 8.21a

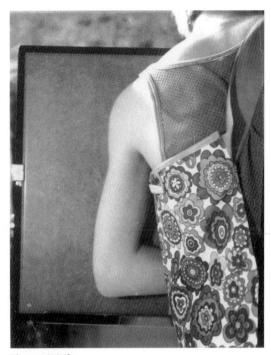

Figure 8.21b

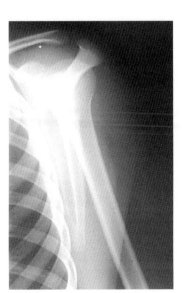

Figure 8.22

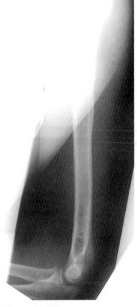

Figure 8.23

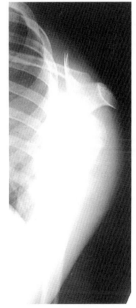

Figure 8.24

**Humerus: diaphysis**

■ Fractures are much less common than in adults and constitute only 2% of all paediatric fractures (Rockwood *et al.*, 1996).

■ Rare under 10 years of age; suspect NAI if under 3 years of age.

■ The fracture is usually complete. It is not manipulated; it is reduced by gravity in a collar-and-cuff sling.

■ Therefore only one AP view is taken at first, if it shows a fracture (Fig. 8.25).

■ The standard two views are taken (erect) within days, to show reduction (Fig. 8.26).

■ If supine on a stretcher, the child should be carefully sat up, with legs over the side of the stretcher, and positioned erect at chest stand. This causes less disturbance to the arm than inserting a cassette under the supine patient.

■ If the arm is immobilized in a J plaster, the lateral view needs increased exposure to penetrate the double thickness of plaster (Fig. 8.27).

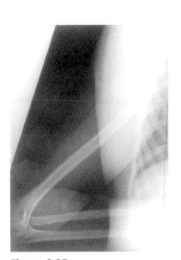

Figure 8.25

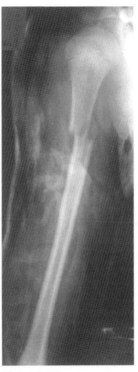

Figure 8.26a

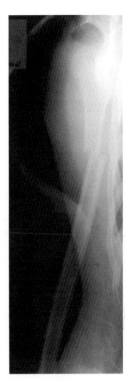

Figure 8.26b

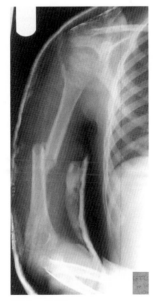

Figure 8.27a

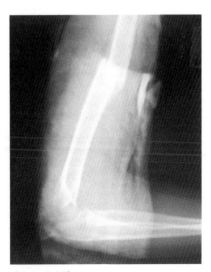

Figure 8.27b

**Elbow region**

- If the request is for 'humerus and elbow', only the lower half of the humerus should be included for either view. Figure 8.28 shows a supracondylar fracture in a 6-year-old, which is almost off the film.

- In children younger than 3 years of age, by far the commonest injury is 'pulled elbow', with negative x-ray findings. A sharp pull jerks the radial head out of the annular ligament.

- In the age range of 3–4 years, the most likely injury is a greenstick supracondylar fracture or fractured lateral condyle, therefore an **AP view of the lower humerus,** not of the elbow joint, is needed if the extension is limited (Fig. 8.29).

- Over 4 years of age, other metaphyseal/epiphyseal fractures occur, at the distal humerus or proximal radius and ulna.

- If the suspected injury is not specified on the request form, two AP views are recommended (Fig. 8.30) and a lateral, if the child cannot fully extend the arm. It is essential to have a true AP view of the **fracture** not the elbow joint.

- An 'equal angles' AP view makes diagnosis impossible (Thornton and Gyll, 1983).

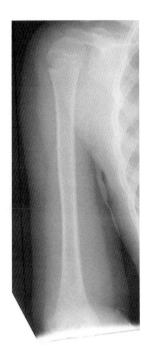

Figure 8.28

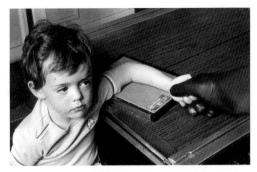

Figure 8.29a

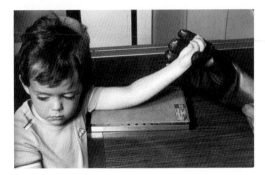

Figure 8.29b

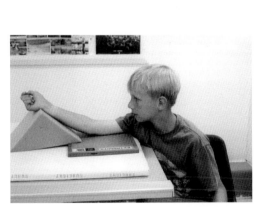

Figure 8.30a

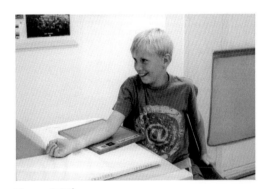

Figure 8.30b

- The standard positioning with vertical beam projection should not be used unless the child can put his or her own arm on the x-ray table and rotate/extend it for the AP view.

- The shoulder and elbow must be in the same plane to give a true lateral view; not always easy with small children.

- True AP/lateral views may be more easily achieved by positioning the child at chest stand for horizontal beam projection.

- It is possible to do this even with a child as young as 2 years of age (Figs 8.31, 8.32). External rotation for a lateral view is shown in Fig. 8.32. Each child was seated on a special paediatric seat at a chest stand and held or supported by a parent. Both were 2 years old.

- Horizontal beam projection at the chest stand should be first choice for imaging any swollen, painful elbow.

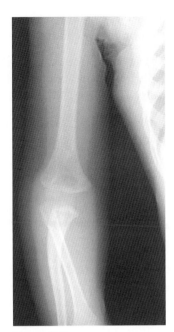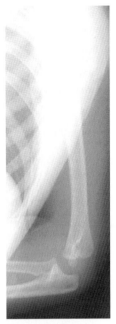

Figure 8.31a

Figure 8.31b

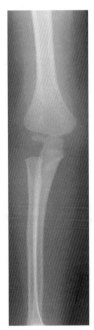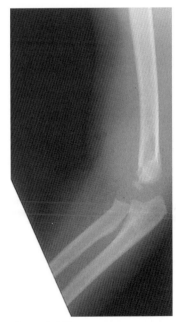

Figure 8.32a

Figure 8.32b

***Supracondylar fracture***

■ The most common injury of the elbow region, peaking at age 4–8 years. It is much more common in children than in adults.

■ There is a wide range of severity, from barely visible undisplaced or greenstick to gross displacement of a complete fracture. It presents in any degree of flexion/extension from 90° to 180°.

■ The elbow should be x-rayed in the presenting position: flexion or extension is equally dangerous if a fracture is present.

■ The age and condition of the child determines the positioning technique.

■ A crying frightened 4- or 5-year-old child is best sitting at a chest stand, not at the x-ray table, for a horizontal beam technique using two separate cassettes.

■ A co-operative 7- or 8-year-old could try standard positioning but if this is painful transfer the child to the chest stand.

■ A 9-year-old in position for an AP view of the lower humerus using horizontal beam projection is shown in Fig. 8.33.

■ For a mediolateral view the child supports the forearm in full supination (Fig. 8.34a) before turning to face the cassette (Fig. 8.34b and c).

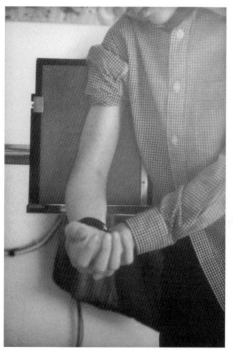

Figure 8.33a

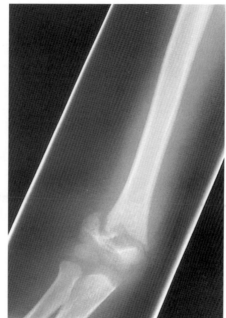

Figure 8.33b

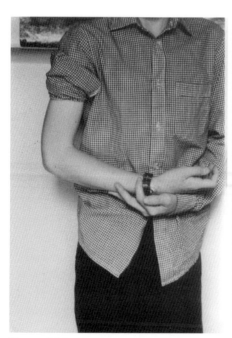

Figure 8.34a

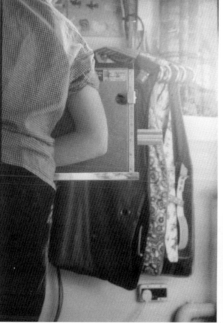

Figure 8.34b

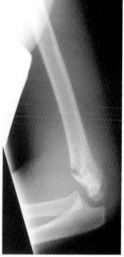

Figure 8.34c

■ A swollen, painful, deformed elbow could be either a severely displaced supracondylar fracture (Fig. 8.35) or dislocation (uncommon; Fig. 8.36). Clinically, they look alike.

■ The standard two views are not needed for diagnosis: one lateral view is enough (Thornton & Gyll, 1999). This should be the agreed protocol in all A & E departments.

■ The lateral view is preferred because it gives more information, is less hazardous to a child's arm and is less difficult to position accurately.

■ An AP view can be taken in theatre under general anaesthetic when the arm can be more safely positioned by the orthopaedic surgeon.

*NOTE* An AP view taken before reduction with the elbow in extreme flexion is mistakenly advocated in some UK textbooks. This is the post-reduction position.

### Common faults

■ The result of an inappropriate request is seen in Fig. 8.37. The x-ray request was for 'Elbow, forearm and wrist'.

■ Underexposure: if much soft tissue swelling is present, exposure factors need to be increased.

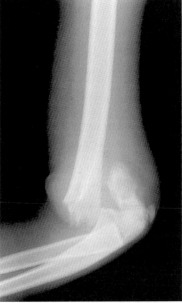

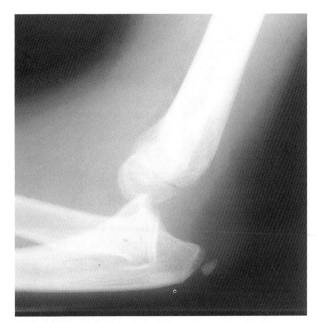

Figure 8.35

Figure 8.36

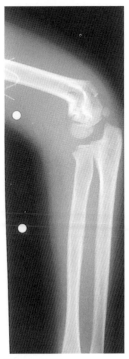

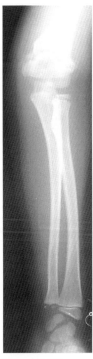

Figure 8.37a

Figure 8.37b

**Post-reduction**

- An AP view in full flexion, positioned by the surgeon in theatre (Fig. 8.38). An increase in exposure of at least 10 kV is required.

- Usually set in a collar-and-cuff sling, perhaps with plaster back slab.

- Position for an AP view in collar-and-cuff sling (Fig. 8.39).

- The horizontal x-ray beam must be very accurately centred, and angled parallel to the upper surface of the forearm, or the result will be as in Fig. 8.40a.

- Figure 8.40b shows that this view can be achieved even with the added difficulty of a plaster back slab.

- If the elbow is set in greater flexion, the x-ray beam needs to be centred through the forearm, with an increase in exposure of 10–15 kV.

- The position for a lateral view in a collar-and-cuff sling is shown in Fig. 8.41. The child needs to lean towards the injured arm, to separate it away from the body, perhaps holding the chest stand with the other hand.

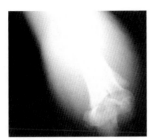

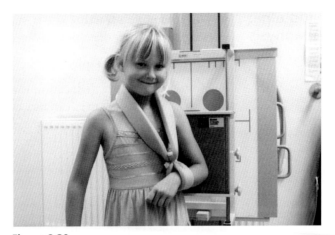

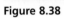

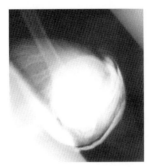

**Figure 8.38**

**Figure 8.39**

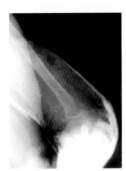

**Figure 8.40a**

**Figure 8.40b**

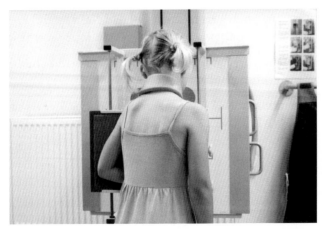

**Figure 8.41**

**Radius and ulna: diaphysis**

■ The commonest fracture site is midshaft, greenstick or complete. It occurs in school-age children (aged 5 years and over).

■ For radius/ulna metaphyseal fractures, see 'Wrist', p. 160.

■ Monteggia fracture dislocation is rare, school age and adolescence occurs. Some paediatric variants exist. If an isolated proximal ulna fracture is seen on forearm films, a localized lateral view of the elbow is needed.

■ A midshaft fracture of one bone only will have an associated proximal or distal joint displacement, needing AP or PA and lateral views of both joints.

■ The choice of positioning and projection is determined by whether or not pain is caused. If a fracture is present, attempts at standard positioning with a vertical beam projection will cause unjustified pain, usually resulting in two oblique views. Figure 8.42 shows this common fault of incorrect positioning. (Note that the adult's fingers are irradiated.)

■ It is very important that both views are 'true' (i.e. accurate). A PA view and horizontal beam lateral view cause least pain and give best results.

■ If a lateral view is taken first, the PA view can be taken on the other half of the same film, avoiding the common practice of reversing the cassette.

■ Young children (less than 5 years old) should not be laid on the x-ray table. They can sit on a parent's lap or stand. Figure 8.43 shows a 3-year-old in position.

■ The child's hand must be held for a lateral view, to prevent it rotating forward, causing an oblique view (Fig. 8.44a).

■ The correct positioning of a 1-year-old child is shown in Fig. 8.44b, resulting in lateral view Fig 8.44c.

■ Midshaft fractures are unusual under 5 years of age; suspicious of an NAI if under 1 year old.

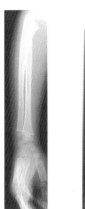 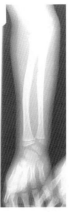

Figure 8.42a    Figure 8.42b

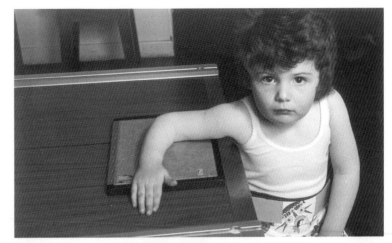

Figure 8.43a

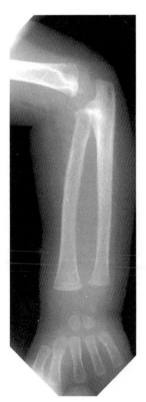

Figure 8.43b

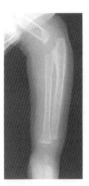

Figure 8.44a

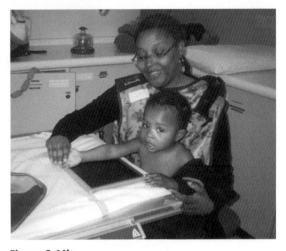

Figure 8.44b

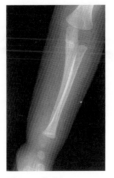

Figure 8.44c

***Post-reduction***

■ The elbow is immobilized at right angles in plaster of Paris. The forearm may be in pronation, supination or, most commonly, halfway between. Post-reduction radiographs are usually taken in Recovery.

■ Position for a PA view (Fig. 8.45a) and horizontal beam lateral view (Fig 8.45b) if the child is prone.

■ Position for AP (Fig. 8.46a) and lateral view (Fig. 8.46b) if the child is supine.

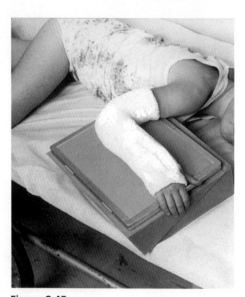

**Figure 8.45a**

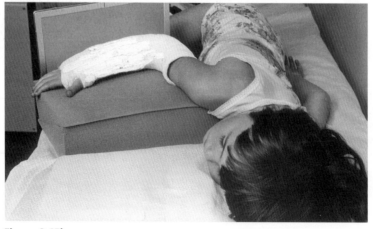

**Figure 8.45b**

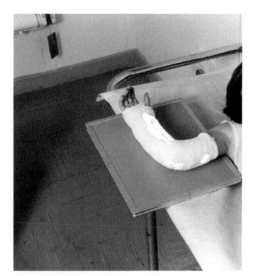

**Figure 8.46a**

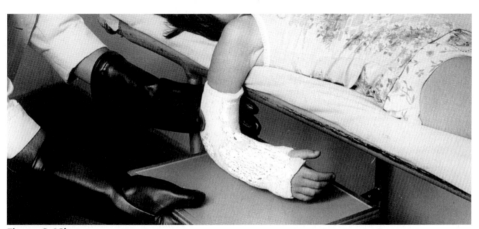

**Figure 8.46b**

■ An 18-month-old toddler in Recovery (Fig. 8.47): arm positioned for a horizontal beam lateral view, with the mother holding the child's elbow. AP or PA view can be taken with vertical beam projection, with the arm and cassette on the trolley (as in Fig. 8.46a).

■ AP and lateral views are taken with a horizontal beam when the forearm is immobilized in **supination**.

■ Positioning for the AP view (Fig. 8.48a) and for the lateral view (Fig. 8.48b). Note in (b) the doubled lead rubber behind the cassette, and foam wedge to keep the cassette vertical.

■ These positions can also be used when the forearm is set in **pronation**.

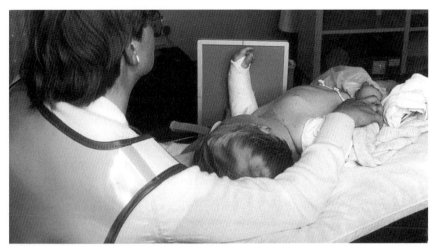

Figure 8.47

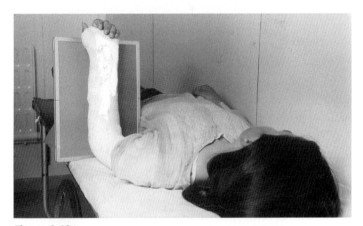

Figure 8.48a

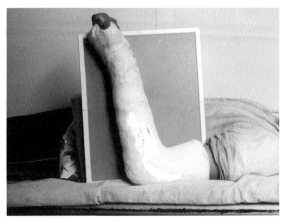

Figure 8.48b

***Follow-up in the fracture clinic***

Forearm set in **halfway position:**

■ A child sitting at the x-ray table for a PA view, with vertical beam projection (Fig. 8.49).

■ The child then stands to get the arm in position for a vertical beam lateral view. However, this is impossible as the child's head will always be in the way (try it for yourself) and the view will be oblique if the head is moved out of the way (Fig. 8.50a).

■ Figure 8.50b shows a repeat lateral view (same child as in Fig. 8.50a) with a horizontal beam projection.

■ Positioning (Fig. 8.51). If this view is taken first, a PA view with vertical projection can be taken on the other half of the film.

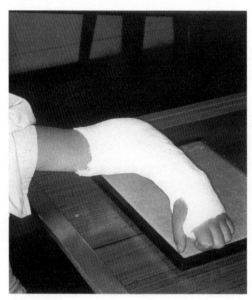

**Figure 8.49**

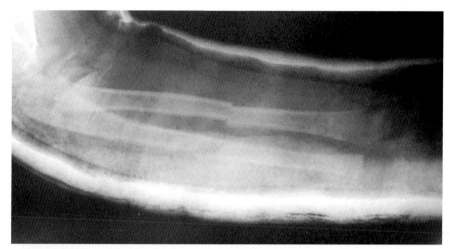

Figure 8.50a

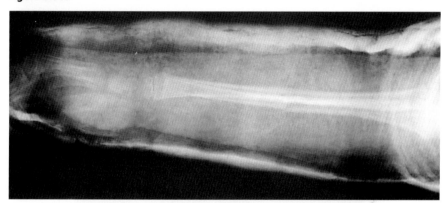

Figure 8.50b

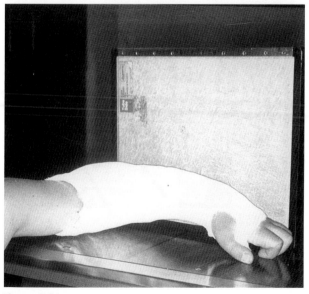

Figure 8.51

Forearm set in **supination:**

■ A 12-year-old girl standing at a chest stand for a horizontal beam lateral view (Fig. 8.52). Note the paediatric lead apron.

■ A 7-year-old boy positioned at the x-ray table for an AP view with vertical beam projection (Fig. 8.53a): 45° foam pad under the armpit and the boy is leaning towards the side of the injured arm.

■ The position for a lateral view with horizontal beam projection (Fig. 8.53b). The boy's shoulder is lower than the forearm to achieve a true lateral view.

Forearm set in pronation:

■ The position for an AP view (Fig. 8.54a) with the boy sitting on a low stool (or a child's chair from the waiting room).

■ The position for a lateral view (Fig. 8.54b). The thumb side of the forearm is on the cassette with the shoulder slightly lower than the table top to achieve a true lateral view.

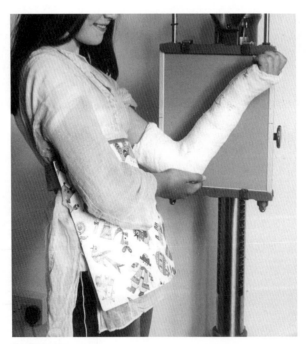

**Figure 8.52**

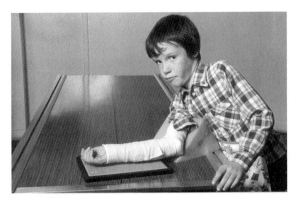

Figure 8.53a

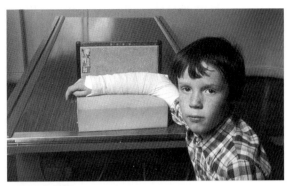

Figure 8.53b

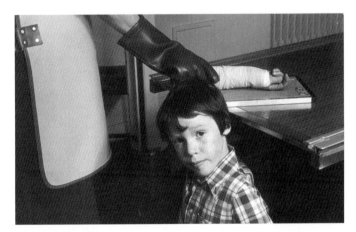

Figure 8.54a

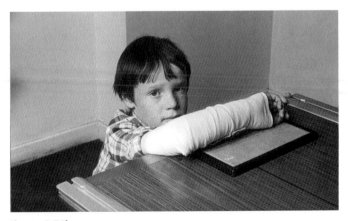

Figure 8.54b

**The wrist**
- Wrist injuries are almost entirely metaphyseal fractures of the radius and ulna. They are very common after infancy and constitute 80% of forearm fractures.

- Request forms usually ask for 'forearm and wrist' or 'wrist and hand' with provisional diagnosis of a scaphoid or Colles' fracture (adult injuries).

- If symptoms are confined to the wrist, only the distal third of the radius/ulna shafts should be included. Fingers should not be x-rayed if uninjured.

- Scaphoid fracture does not occur until about 12 years of age, and is rare then. Scaphoid views should not be taken under that age even if requested.

- Juvenile Colles' fracture is an epiphyseal injury: fracture separation of the radial epiphysis, occurring only at approximately 6–12 years of age (Fig. 8.55).

- Distal metaphyseal fractures may be buckle, greenstick or complete, of both bones or of the radius alone; commonly complete radius and greenstick ulna fractures.

- If clinical deformity is present, or movement causes pain, horizontal beam projection should be used for the lateral view (Fig. 8.56).

- Complete fracture of the distal radial metaphysis in isolation is a well-known paediatric entity (Fig. 8.57). Routine extra views of the whole forearm, to look for an associated upper ulnar fracture, are not needed if the cause of injury was a simple fall on outstretched hand.

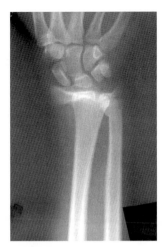

Figure 8.55a

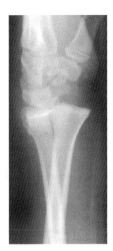

Figure 8.55b

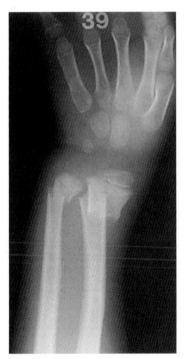

Figure 8.56a

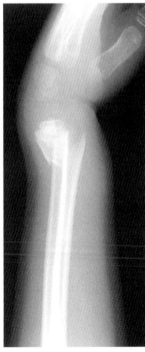

Figure 8.56b

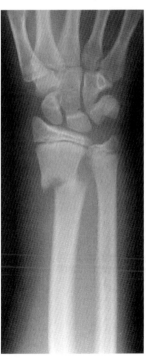

Figure 8.57

- A 3-year-old girl standing by the x-ray table (Fig. 8.58). For the lateral view, the child's hand must be held tilted dorsally by a parent.

- A 1- or 2-year-old can sit on the mother's lap (Fig. 8.59). Again, the hand is tilted dorsally for the lateral view.

*Common faults*

- Under-exposure: if much soft tissue swelling is present, the exposure factors need to be increased.

- Over-exposure: if plaster is only a back slab (Fig. 8.60), the exposure factors need to be decreased.

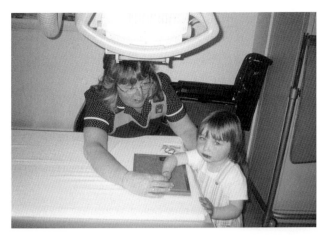

Figure 8.58

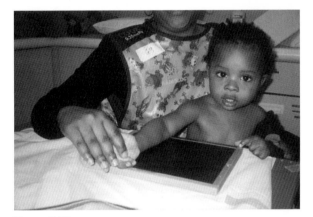

Figure 8.59

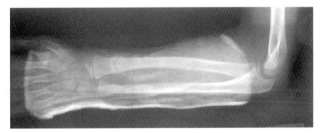

Figure 8.60a

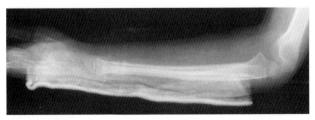

Figure 8.60b

**The hand**

■ Hand injuries are much less common than in adults. The usual causes are sports injuries in teenagers, fighting amongst schoolboys and toddlers' fingers trapped in doors.

■ If a phalangeal fracture is seen on the standard oblique view of hand, an extra lateral view of the finger is essential.

■ A 2-year-old girl seated sideways to the x-ray table on her mother's lap (Fig. 8.61).

■ A 3-year-old can kneel on a stool or stand at the x-ray table (Fig. 8.62).

■ Older children are x-rayed as adults.

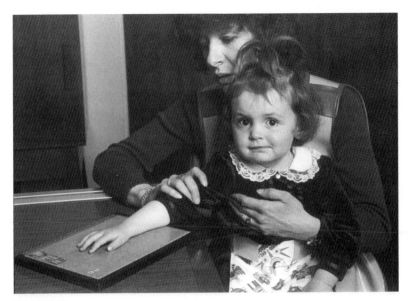

Figure 8.61

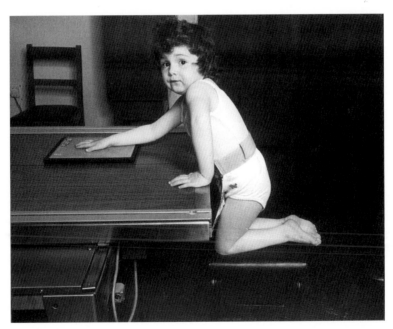

Figure 8.62

■ The hand and wrist of a baby is x-rayed for a bone age estimate, seldom for injury.

■ Figure 8.63 shows a 3-month-old baby positioned prone with a Bucky-band immobilizing the pelvis/legs, with her hand immobilized under a strip of clear film or Dycem (an effective alternative).

■ Both hands together for an orthopaedic condition, congenital deformity, etc. Should be taken with the child standing away from the x-ray table and leaning forwards for maximum distance as gonad protection (Fig. 8.64). It is very difficult to get comparative PA views if the child is sitting sideways to the x-ray table.

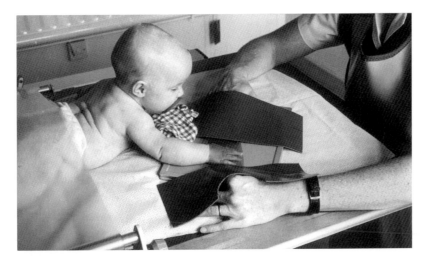

Figure 8.63

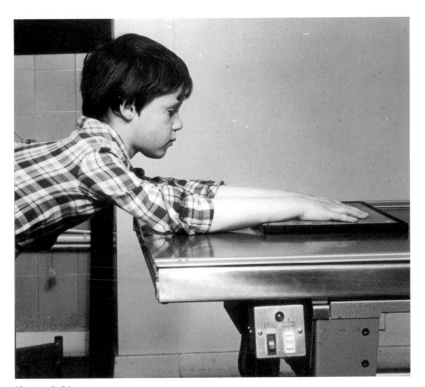

Figure 8.64

# 9 The leg

**Hip**

- Hip fracture or dislocation is very rare in isolation, usually seen only as part of severe pelvic disruption.

- If a lateral view of one hip is necessary, the 'frog' positioning of both hips (Fig. 9.1a) is used, with the child off-centred and the beam collimated to the hip in question (Fig. 9.1b). Gonad protection must be very carefully placed.

- In the standard positioning for a lateral view (45° rotation of the pelvis to the affected side with hip and knee flexed) gonad protection of boys is impossible (Fig. 9.2) and of girls very difficult.

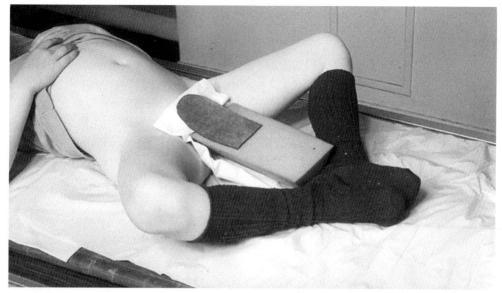

Figure 9.1a

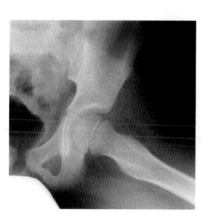

Figure 9.1b

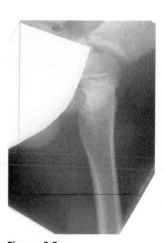

Figure 9.2a

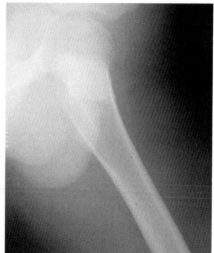

Figure 9.2b

There are three specifically paediatric conditions involving the hip.

**Developmental dysplasia of the hip (DDH, formerly CDH)**

■ Female to male proportion is 5:1.

■ Infants are clinically screened at birth for hip stability. If doubtful, they are treated in double nappies or a Pavlic harness (Fig. 9.3), and checked with sonography at 4–6 weeks.

■ The first x-ray examination is not until 3–4 months of age: the capital epiphysis is not visible until then. AP view only, with legs straight and feet together (Fig. 9.4). The mother's hands are unprotected here to show how the legs are held. A lead rubber 'arch' cut-out should be used (see also Fig. 10.3, p. 215).

■ This view is repeated at intervals, if necessary, for follow-up. Figure 9.5 shows a 2-year-old girl positioned.

■ The 'frog-leg' lateral view (abduction and external rotation, flexed knees) and von Rosen view (45° abduction, internal rotation) are not taken. Positioning for either demonstrates reduction rather than the presence of subluxation. The von Rosen view was intended only for neonates.

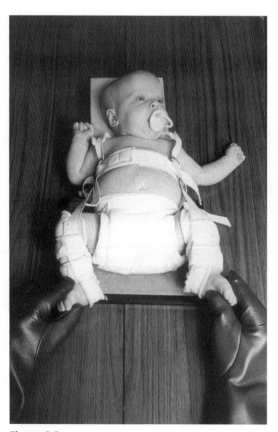

**Figure 9.3**

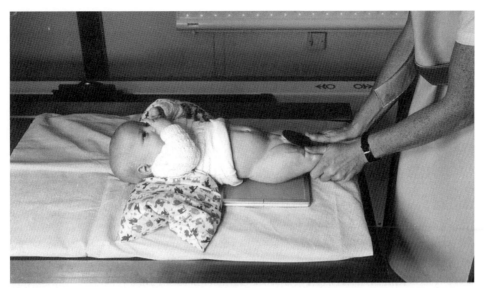

Figure 9.4

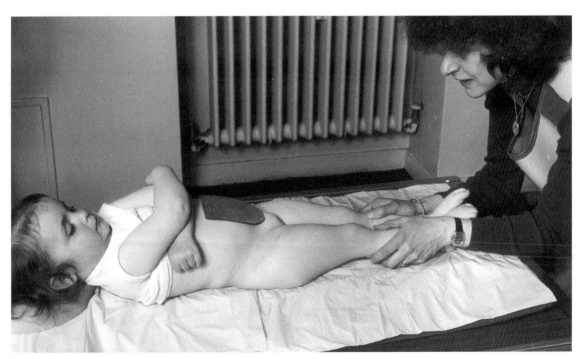

Figure 9.5

■ Further treatment includes closed reduction under general anaesthetic, and immobilization in a hip spica (Fig. 9.6). Computed tomography, or in some centres zonography, demonstrates the hip through plaster. Gonad dose is high.

■ Cases of late diagnosis, or unsuccessful treatment, may have open reduction and Salter's (pelvic) osteotomy or femoral derotation osteotomy. Both are immobilized in, and x-rayed through, hip spicas.

### Common faults

■ The pelvis not being level (Fig. 9.7). Compare correct position (a) with rotated (b). The criterion is that both obturator foramina should be equally open.

■ Inaccurate positioning of gonad protection (see p. 179).

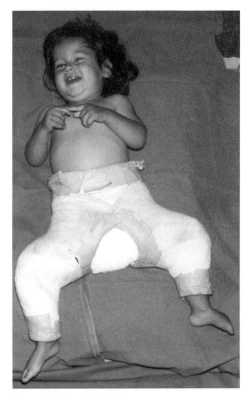

Figure 9.6

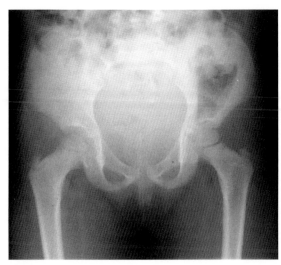

Figure 9.7a

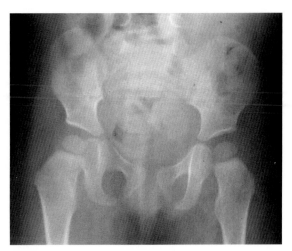

Figure 9.7b

**Perthes'
(Legg–Calvé–
Perthes) disease**

■ The condition is usually idiopathic; interrupted blood supply to the femoral head epiphysis leading to vascular necrosis and dislocation if untreated. The male to female proportion is 5:1, peak age 4–8 years.

■ Positioning for an AP view of both hips is as for DDH (Fig. 9.8). A sandbag against the 5-year-old's ankles to keep feet together and ankles aligned.

■ Positioning for 'frog' lateral view: abduction, and external rotation with the soles of the feet together (Fig. 9.9); 45° foam pads may be needed to support the knees. Note the use of a small 45° pad under gonad protection.

■ Clinical check monthly, re-x-ray perhaps 6-monthly, for signs of dislocation of deforming femoral head. Surgical treatment will possibly be required.

■ Hand is x-rayed for bone age, which is often delayed.

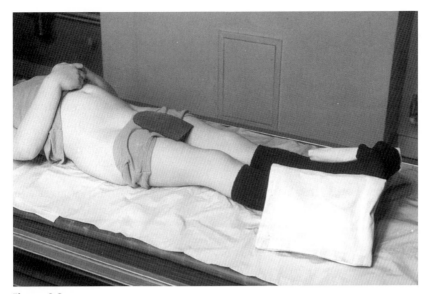

Figure 9.8

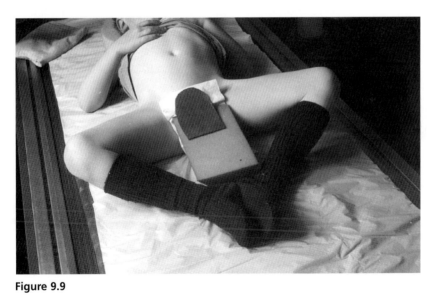

Figure 9.9

**Slipped capital femoral epiphysis (SCFE)**

■ Usually of slow onset but may present acutely after a fall.

■ Occurs at 10–15 or 16 years of age, which is a period of rapid growth and mostly in obese children.

■ AP view of both hips is taken, as for the previous conditions (Fig. 9.10a). A lateral view is essential on first examination (Fig. 9.10b). Diagnosis can be missed on an AP view alone.

■ A horizontal beam lateral view is standard but gives a greater gonad dose.

■ A 'frog' lateral view is preferred by some as it gives a lower gonad dose but this positioning may be impossible due to pain.

■ Treatment is pinning with one to three Steinmann pins, which are removed a year later. Some surgeons also pin the normal hip prophylactically.

**Gonad protection**

■ It is remarkable how often gonad protection is misplaced or of inadequate shape.

■ Correct placing is shown in Fig. 9.11: (a) girl; (b) boy. In some centres it is omitted on the first film of a baby girl with DDH, and on both boys and girls in A & E departments. 'Figure of Eight' gonad protection is shown in Fig. 9.11c.

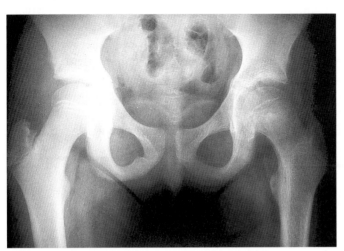

Figure 9.10a

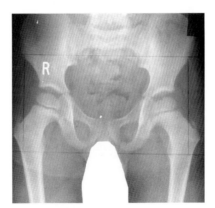

Figure 9.10b

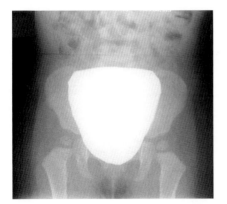

Figure 9.11a

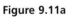

Figure 9.11b

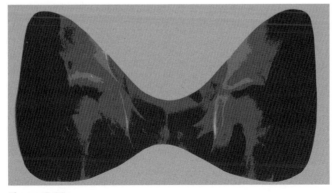

Figure 9.11c

- A variety of mistaken placings seen in Figs 9.12–9.14.
  - Figure 9.12 shows overenthusiastic wrapping of a baby's scrotum, which has left his testes uncovered.
  - Boys' underpants should be pulled down so that the waist elastic is over the symphysis pubis, and a lead shield placed over the testes. In Fig. 9.13 the testes are over the symphysis pubis because the underpants have not been pulled down. It is impossible to balance the gonad shield in place.
  - Figures 9.14 and 9.15 show completely inadequate shapes and sizes of lead protection.
  - Figure 9.16 shows indecision as to whether the patient is a boy or girl....
  - Figure 9.17 is a girl!

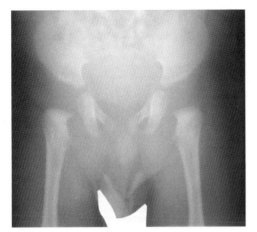

Figure 9.12

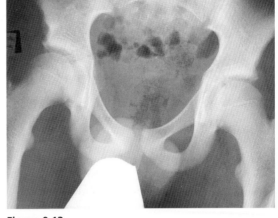

Figure 9.13

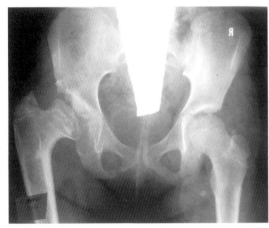

Figure 9.14

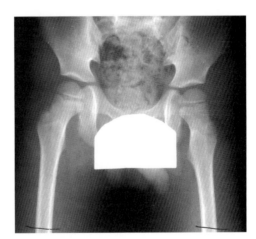

Figure 9.15

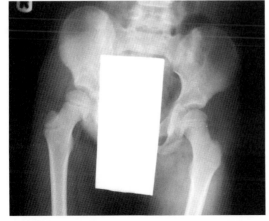

Figure 9.16

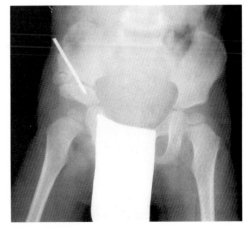

Figure 9.17

**Femur: diaphysis**

■ A midshaft transverse or oblique fracture is almost always complete; this constitutes 70% of femoral fractures. Common at all ages: peak 2–10 years.

■ Less than 2 years of age, usually unsplinted, presents in external rotation with the knee flexed (Fig. 9.18a, b).

■ Positioning for the AP view includes rotation and extension of the leg; this is cruel and unjustified (Fig. 9.18c). Compare with (b).

■ A lateral view in the presenting position is enough if positive.

■ The child is put in 'gallows' traction on the ward and re-x-rayed within 24 hours; both views are taken then (Fig. 9.19).

■ Requests from A & E often specify both legs but this is an unjustified radiation dose.

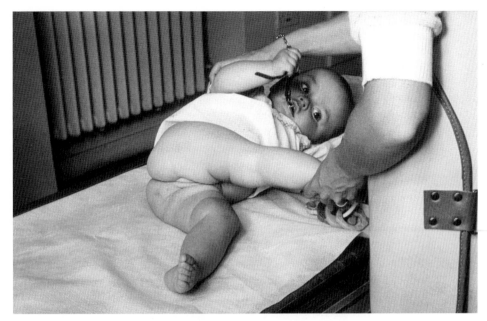

Figure 9.18a

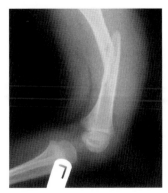

Figure 9.18b

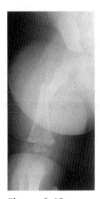

Figure 9.18c

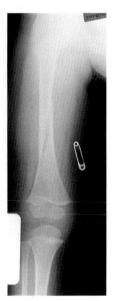

Figure 9.19a

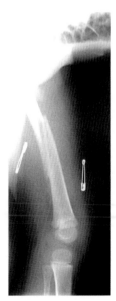

Figure 9.19b

***'Gallows' traction***
■ Fixed traction (Fig. 9.20). This is a portable 'gallows' so that the child can be nursed at home.

■ Sliding traction on an overhead bar (Fig. 9.21); 7-month-old baby lying across the cot.

■ An 18-month-old child in fixed traction on an overhead bar (Fig. 9.22).

■ Note that the pelvis is suspended above the mattress, allowing gravity to increase traction.

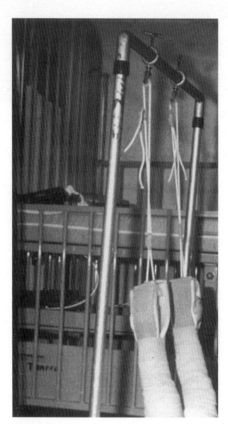

**Figure 9.20**

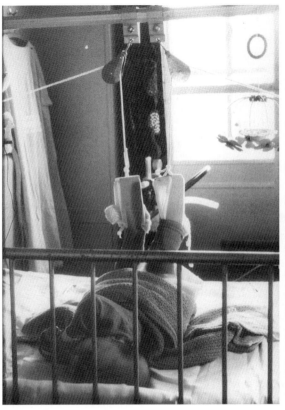

**Figure 9.21**

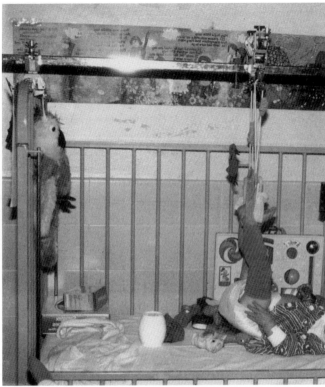

**Figure 9.22**

### Positioning

■ X-ray tube and cassette in position for an AP view (Fig. 9.23a, b) with the beam collimated to the fractured femur only (Fig. 9.23c).

■ The collimator is against the cot bars to project them at maximum distance apart. The central ray must be midway between the bars.

■ Before exposure, the nappy (diaper) should be removed and the child's hands held out of the way.

■ Position for the lateral view with the cot side lowered (Fig. 9.24a). The child is moved slightly towards the end of the cot to avoid the metal upright of the 'gallows'. (This is not necessary with an overhead bar as in Figs 9.21 and 9.22.) The uninjured leg is untied and extended, caudad or cephalad, clear of the fractured leg (Fig. 9.24b).

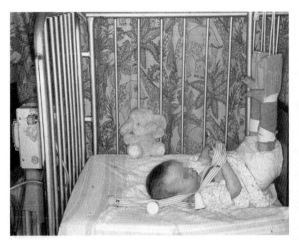

Figure 9.23a

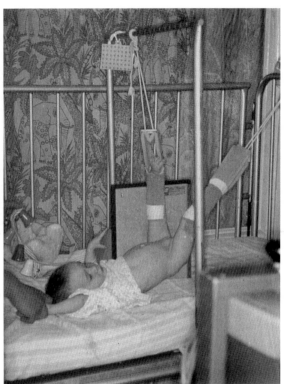

Figure 9.24a

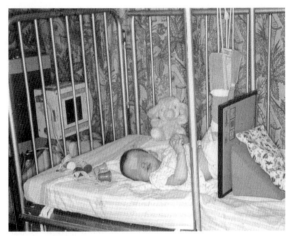

Figure 9.23b

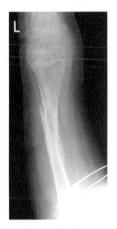

Figure 9.23c

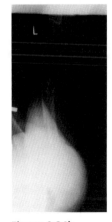

Figure 9.24b

**Common faults**

- Leaving the nappy on: two cases shown in Fig. 9.25.

- Incorrectly placed gonad protection in the same plane as the horizontal x-ray beam, hence the testes are irradiated (Fig. 9.26a). This is the placing for use with the **vertical** beam. Protection must be at right angles to the beam.

- Misplacement of the cassette **between** the legs (Fig. 9.26b). It is possible for half the fracture to be excluded.

- Compare correct placement against the outer aspect of the leg (Fig. 9.26c). This is the same child, one week later (different radiographer).

- Figure 9.26: these radiographs are shown as taken, i.e. with the feet in the air.

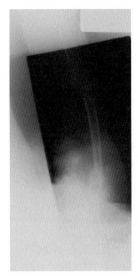
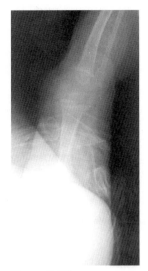

Figure 9.25a                    Figure 9.25b

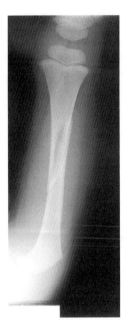
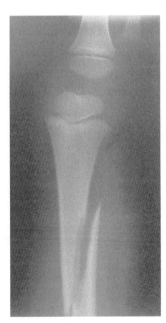
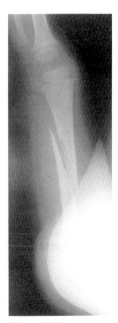

Figure 9.26a                    Figure 9.26b                    Figure 9.26c

***Older child***

- The unsplinted leg lies, like the baby's, in external rotation, with knee flexed.

- The first view to locate the fracture is a lateral, including the hip and knee (Fig. 9.27), a 7-year-old road traffic accident (RTA) victim.

- The second view is centred to the fracture with horizontal beam projection (Fig. 9.28a). **The leg must not be rotated.**

- It is essential to indicate the hip and knee joints on this view. Hip ←, Knee →, must be written on the film.

- Gonad protection is misplaced in Fig. 9.28a but serves to identify the hip end of the femur. Correct protection is shown in Fig. 9.28b: the lead rubber cut-out fits over the thigh.

- A 3-year-old child: another RTA victim (Fig. 9.29a). Knee presenting extended. The second view was taken with a horizontal beam but does not include the proximal end of the fracture (Fig. 9.29b).

- Does it matter? The whole of the femoral shaft could be included only by placing the cassette against the **outer** aspect of the thigh, raising the uninjured leg out of the way and using a mediolateral projection of the beam. However, this may not be considered worthwhile, as there will be no manipulation of the fracture.

- Note that in both of the above cases, muscle pull has rotated the lower fragment by 90°. There is an AP view of the hip and a lateral view of the knee on the same film in each case.

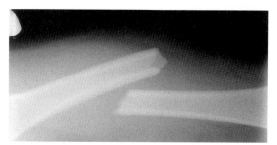

Figure 9.28a

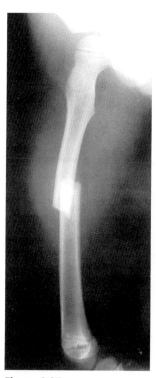

Figure 9.27

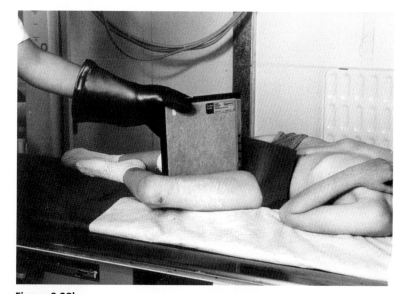

Figure 9.28b

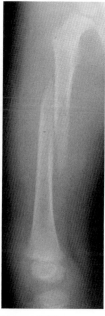

Figure 9.29a

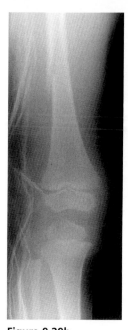

Figure 9.29b

■ Figure 9.30 shows two views of a 6-year-old boy's unsplinted femur. From the presenting position (a) the leg has been turned and the knee straightened for an AP view (b). The upper half of the femur has hardly moved but the lower half has rotated by 90°. **The pivot of rotation is the fracture**. This is condemned as dangerous and cruel.

■ A 5-year-old boy in sliding traction (Fig. 9.31a) is x-rayed as an adult. Very careful placing of the gonad shield is necessary, altered 90° from the AP placement for the horizontal beam second view. The usual placing of the shield as in Fig. 9.31b is useless with horizontal beam projection.

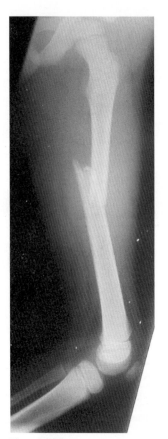
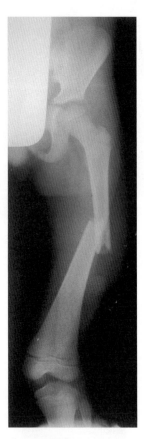

**Figure 9.30a**     **Figure 9.30b**

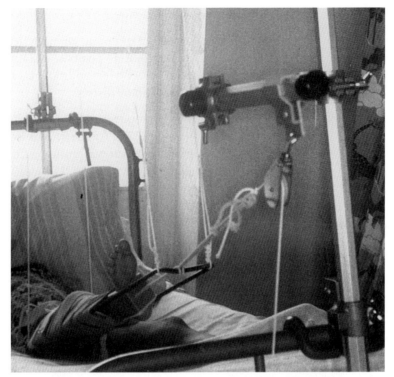

Figure 9.31a

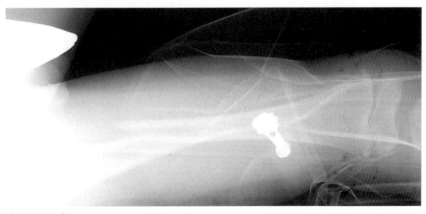

Figure 9.31b

**Femur: distal metaphysis**

A common site for two other fractures:

■ A greenstick or buckle fracture in young children (less than 5 years of age). A lateral view in the presenting position establishes the fracture (Fig. 9.32). It is doubtful if an AP view adds any useful information; it may be omitted if it causes pain or distress.

■ A pathological fracture in osteoporotic disease. A lateral view taken in the presenting position (Fig. 9.33a). As the knee is flexed at 90°, an AP view (b) with a horizontal beam was unsuccessful. (c) The repeat PA view shows the fracture.

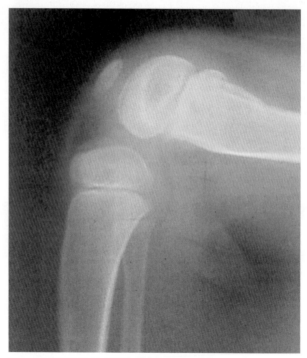

**Figure 9.32**

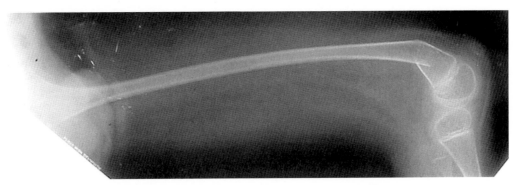

Figure 9.33a

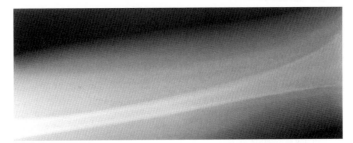

Figure 9.33b

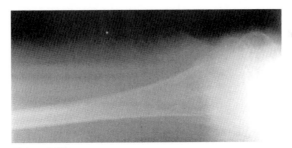

Figure 9.33c

**Knee joint**

- All knee fractures are uncommon, occurring mostly in teenagers. Dislocation is almost unknown.

- A Salter-type epiphyseal fracture separation, distal femur or proximal tibia, are the most likely fractures, caused by sports injury or RTA.

- Avulsion of the tibial spine occurs in children over 5 years of age; avulsion of the tibial tubercle from 13 to 16 years of age; patella injuries are very rare before adolescence.

- The splinted leg is x-rayed as for adults.

- The unsplinted leg presents with a flexed knee. This must not be straightened for an AP view as **extension can damage the popliteal artery**.

- In children less than 5 years old, an x-ray request for 'knee' should always include the whole length of the tibia (see p. 196).

- A lateral view must be 'true' lateral. Even a slightly oblique view can show a misleading appearance of the tibial tubercle as though avulsed (Fig. 9.34). A 15° foam pad under the ankle is recommended.

- Osteochondritis dissecans affects adolescents. A small piece of the articular surface of the medial femoral condyle separates, becoming a loose body in the joint. A tunnel view is needed as well as AP lateral views.

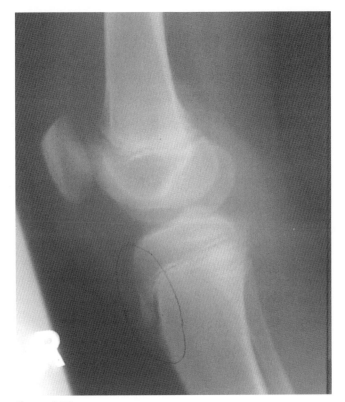

Figure 9.34

**Tibia and fibula: diaphysis**

- Upper shaft fractures are uncommon. The typical fracture site is midshaft or lower third of tibia.

- This is the commonest leg fracture, at all ages, once walking has started. It is usually complete, spiral or oblique. The fibula is often intact.

- The unsplinted leg of a young child presents in external rotation with the knee flexed. A refusal to straighten it or allow manual extension may result in an x-ray request for 'knee'.

- Under 5 years of age, the first view should be a lateral of the whole tibial shaft in the presenting position. Figure 9.35a shows a 3-year-old boy.

- The leg may be rotated for the AP view as movement is at the hip but it is not necessary to extend the knee if distress is caused. A 45° foam pad supports the cassette, with corresponding tube angulation (Fig. 9.35b, c).

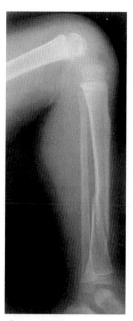

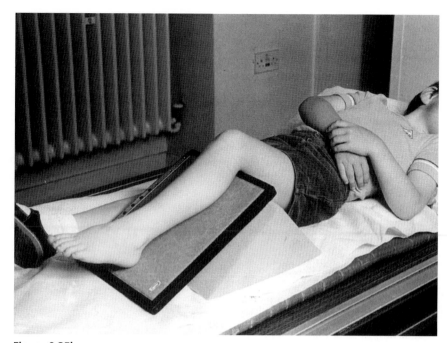

Figure 9.35a

Figure 9.35b

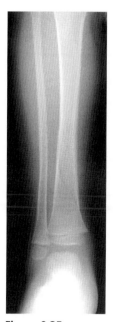

Figure 9.35c

- A fractured tibia presenting in extreme guarding position of the leg (Fig. 9.36a).

- If attempting to rotate the leg causes distress, the AP view is taken with horizontal beam projection (Fig. 9.36b). In Fig. 9.36c, a 3-year-old is shown in position with a 45° foam pad under the opposite buttock, and a small foam pad under the ankle, if possible; align the lower leg with the cassette to get a true AP view.

- Older children (over 6 years of age) will probably be in a splint and are x-rayed as adults.

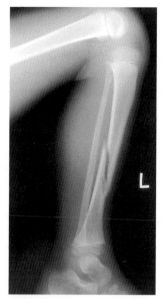

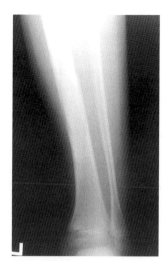

Figure 9.36a

Figure 9.36b

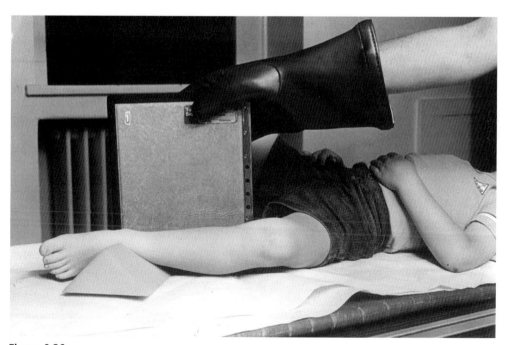

Figure 9.36c

The following case demonstrates the advantage of knowing which fractures are most likely at which ages:

■ A 3-year-old girl arrived in A & E after a fall, lying on a trolley, as seen in Fig. 9.37a: the hip and knee acutely flexed, the knee extending beyond the edge of the trolley. An attempt at clinical examination caused screams of fear. The provisional diagnosis was 'fracture or dislocation of the hip'.

■ The whole of the femoral shaft was x-rayed, as a far more likely site of fracture than the hip. An extra lateral view was taken (Fig. 9.37b) because the lower shaft of the femur was masked by the trolley's edge. Both films were negative.

■ The films were shown to the referring doctor with a request for official permission to move the leg for AP positioning (to reassure the very apprehensive parents). The radiographer also suggested taking a lateral view of the lower leg (the other typical fracture site at this age) before repositioning. The doctor was unconvinced but agreed.

■ This lateral view (Fig. 9.37c) showed a fracture, giving an explanation for the acute 'guarding' position of leg. An AP view was then taken with a horizontal beam projection (Fig. 9.37d).

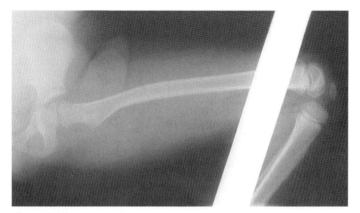

Figure 9.37a

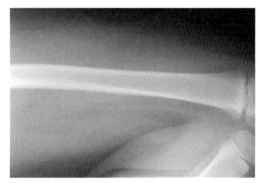

Figure 9.37b

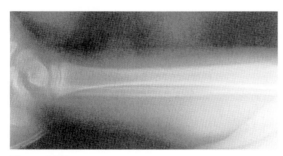

Figure 9.37c

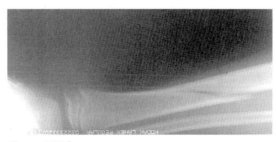

Figure 9.37d

**Toddler's fracture**

- Occurs approximately from 1 to 3 years of age, an undisplaced hairline fracture which is often seen in only one view (Figs 9.38, 9.39).

- In Fig. 9.39b note the careless placing of the cassette: the namespace obscures the ankle.

- Positioning for an AP view of a baby's tibia is almost impossible. Prone positioning for a PA view is more successful (Fig. 9.40). Both legs are held in position with the beam collimated to the injured leg.

- A request for 'whole leg' or 'both legs for comparison' of a toddler who will not weight-bear should be queried with the referring doctor. It should be possible to localize the suspected fracture to the femur or tibia. A routine 'comparison' view is condemned (WHO, 1987).

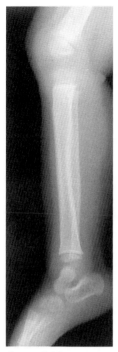

Figure 9.38a

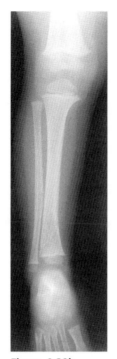

Figure 9.38b

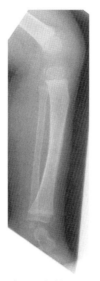

Figure 9.39a

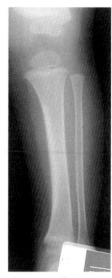

Figure 9.39b

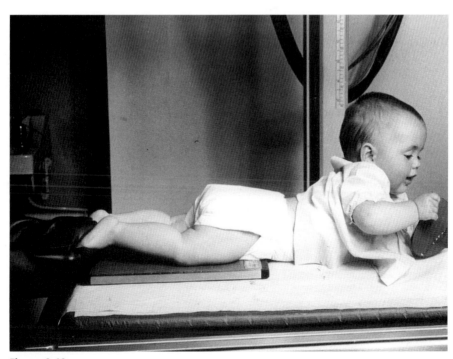

Figure 9.40

**Ankle**

- Buckle fractures of the distal metaphysis are common in babies and toddlers (Fig. 9.41).

- Injuries of the ankle joint in older children involve the epiphysis (Fig. 9.42). Peak age is 9–14 years; this is common.

- Adult Pott's fractures are not seen until after the epiphyses fuse at 16–17 years old.

- X-ray requests for 'ankle and foot' need clarification from the referring doctor as to which is injured.

- The lower third of the tibia should be included when an x-ray request is made for the ankle. However, the whole lower leg should not be x-rayed for a clinically obvious ankle fracture such as Fig. 9.42, as this causes an increased radiation dose.

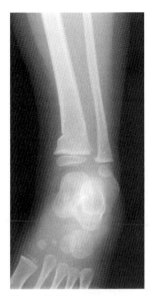

Figure 9.41a

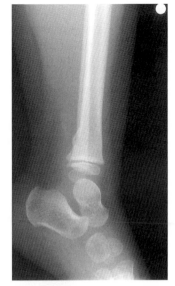

Figure 9.41b

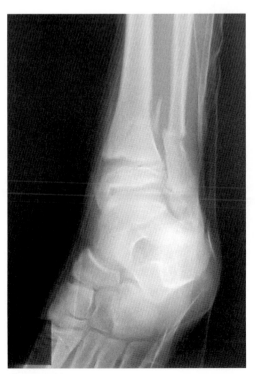

Figure 9.42a

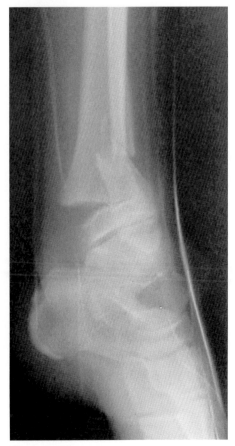

Figure 9.42b

***Common faults***
- In the older child, including the whole shaft of tibia and fibula means gross off-centring of the x-ray beam. The fracture is then distorted or may even be missed. Figure 9.43 shows a distal tibial epiphyseal fracture almost off the edge of the film.

- Omitting to check previous radiographs before a follow-up x-ray examination. Original AP/lateral views are shown in Fig. 9.44a, b. The follow-up lateral view (Fig. 9.44c) almost excludes the fracture site because of the request for 'tibia/fibula'.

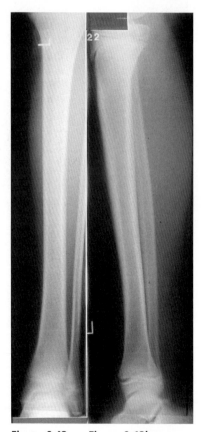

**Figure 9.43a    Figure 9.43b**

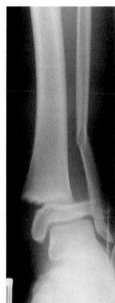
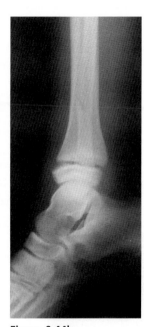
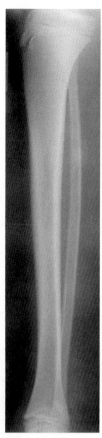
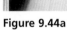

**Figure 9.44a**          **Figure 9.44b**          **Figure 9.44c**

- A buckle fracture in a 12-year-old boy (Fig. 9.45). This is unusual in older children. Inaccurately positioned lateral view: the leg has not been rotated enough nor the knee flexed.

- For minor ankle injuries (sprains, etc.), a true lateral view is easier to achieve with internal rotation (Gyll & Blake, 1986) (Fig. 9.46).

- This positioning is much easier with children than with older patients (Fig. 9.47).

- Young children (less than 5 years of age) should not be made to lie down (as they often are) for ankle or lower leg radiography (Fig. 9.48).

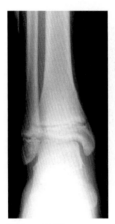

Figure 9.45a

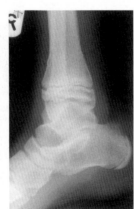

Figure 9.45b

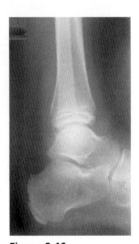

Figure 9.46

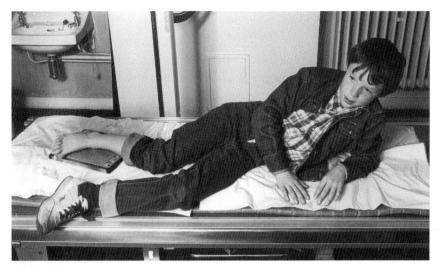

Figure 9.47

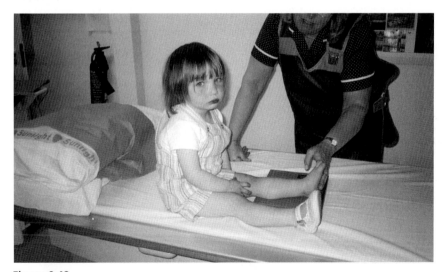

Figure 9.48

**Foot**
- Injuries are uncommon. Metatarsal fractures occur in older children, phalangeal fractures at any age.

- Tarsal injuries are rare. Calcaneal fracture occurs in adolescents: lateral and axial views are taken as for adults.

- Exposure factors and collimation must be appropriate for the injured area, i.e. the fore- or hindfoot.

- Figure 9.49 shows that a clinically obvious toe injury does not need the whole foot to be x-rayed.

- Requests for 'foot and ankle' need clarification from referring doctor as to which is injured.

- Tarsal coalition causes painful flat foot in teenagers. The abnormal cartilaginous bar between the tarsal bones ossifies over time. A dorsiplantar view, collimated to the tarsal area, and a Harris axial projection are appropriate (Stripp, 1979).

- Young children should be x-rayed sitting up, not supine. The baby (Fig. 9.50) and the 2-year-old (Fig. 9.51) sitting on a box feel more secure. The supine position causes anxiety and the child feels more vulnerable.

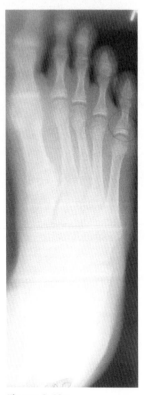

**Figure 9.49a**

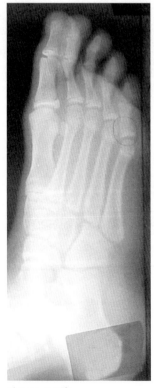

**Figure 9.49b**

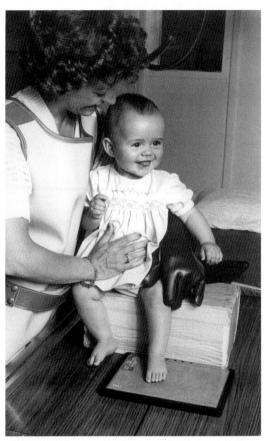

**Figure 9.50**

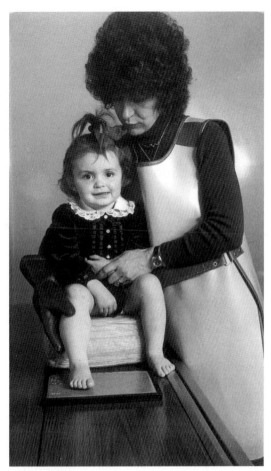

**Figure 9.51**

# 10 Non-accidental injury

**Introduction**

- Non-accidental injury (NAI) can be physical or mental injury, sexual abuse or exploitation, negligence or maltreatment of a child by a person who is responsible for the child's welfare. NAI has an intentional element.

- Skeletal surveys are carried out only at the request of a consultant paediatrician or radiologist, after admission of the child. It is not done from A & E because:
  - Junior doctors may not be competent to diagnose subtle radiological or clinical signs, and may request unnecessarily.
  - A radiographer who is specially trained in paediatric radiography techniques should perform skeletal surveys (British Society for Paediatric Radiology). This is vital for optimization of image quality.

- The need for a survey should be explained to parents beforehand by the paediatrician, so that radiographers are not asked the reason. Parents or carers should be allowed to accompany the child during the examination provided that they have received a full explanation as to why the examination is taking place and as long as their presence does not distress the child.

- Two radiographers working together is recommended because:
  - it speeds up the examination
  - each is a witness to what the other has done (in case of later accusations).

- The radiographers must:
  - maintain a professional non-judgemental attitude during the examination
  - remember that abuse is only suspected at this time
  - control the situation and give clear, concise instructions to the parents/carers.

- Notes must be taken (at the time that the skeletal survey is performed) of who was present, what happened and when it was done. These records should be confidential and stored within the radiology department.

- Special care should be taken to ensure that the films are not mislaid or lost. It is good practice for all films to be duplicated and each set stored in different places.

**Skeletal survey protocols**

- Babygrams **are not** acceptable as the image quality is poor and the radiation dose is much higher than that received from separate films.

- High quality images are essential because of possible legal implications.

- Images must be identified accurately, with no doubt that they belong to the child being x-rayed. The child's name, ensuring correct spelling, should be double-checked. All demographic details should be placed on the film at the time of the examination, either photographically or electronically. It is good practice for both radiographers to sign the name label on each radiograph.

- Orientation markers must be placed on the film at the time of examination so that they are visible. They must not be added later.

- Good bony detail and soft tissue detail must be seen on all images, using a single exposure.

- Eight films is a basic minimum. Note immobilization with a foam pad under the Bucky band in each position:
  - AP view of the chest and humeri (Fig. 10.1). Note the 15° foam pad behind the head to cushion the edge of the cassette and to raise the chin.
  - AP view of the forearms (Fig. 10.2) on separate films.
  - AP view of the pelvis and femora (Fig. 10.3). Note the lead rubber cut-out over the holder's hands. It is very difficult to hold the feet or hands accurately in gloves.
  - PA view of the knees and tibiae (Fig. 10.4).
  - AP/lateral views of the skull (see Chapter 6).
- An extra lateral view is taken of any positive finding.
- Hall (in Carty *et al.*, 1994) adds a lateral dorsilumbar spine and the whole cervical spine.
- In 2003 the British Society for Paediatric Radiology published a Draft Standard for skeletal surveys in suspected non-accidental injuries of children. Their suggested views are:

- *Skull* (SXR)
  - AP and lateral plus Towne's view for occipital injury
  - Skull x-rays should be taken even if a CT scan has been performed

- *Body*
  - AP/frontal chest (including clavicles)
  - Oblique views of ribs (left and right)
  - AP of abdomen with pelvis and hips

- *Spine*
  - Lateral – cervical and thoraco-lumbar

- *Limbs*
  - AP humeri, AP forearms
  - AP femora, AP tibia and fibulae
  - PA hands, AP feet

- Supplemented by:
  - Lateral views of any suspected shaft fracture
  - Lateral coned views of the elbows/wrists/knees/ankles may demonstrate metaphyseal injuries in greater detail than AP views of limbs alone.

- American lists may also include lateral view of chest.

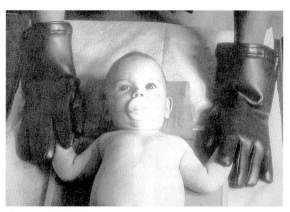

Figure 10.1

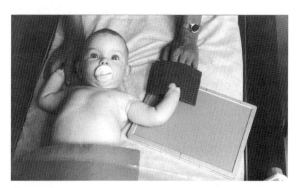

Figure 10.2

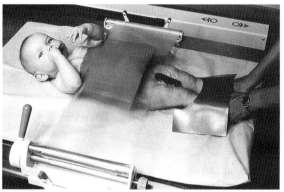

Figure 10.3

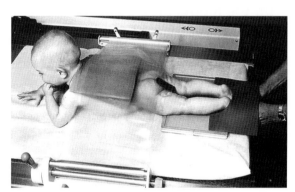

Figure 10.4

# 11 The rights of the child

**Introduction**

There have been significant events that have influenced children's rights within health care environments in the UK.

**United Nations (UN) Convention on the Rights of the Child (United Nations, 1989)**

- This was ratified by the British Government in 1991 and reported to the UN committee in 1994 and 1999.

- It provides a set of principles and minimum standards against which to test law, policy and practice as it affects children and young people.

- Children have three main rights:
  - Non-discrimination, whatever race, sex, language, disability, opinion, family background the child may have.
  - Best interest. When adults or organizations make decisions which affect children, they must always think first about what is best for the child.
  - Children's views must be taken into consideration. What they say must be listened to carefully.
  - Other rights include privacy, access to information, being kept safe from harm, not being separated from their parents against their will (unless it is in the interest of the child), and disabled children must be helped to be as independent as possible.

**The Children Act (WHO, 1989)**

The main principles are that:

- Welfare of the child is paramount.

- Parents with children in need should be helped to bring up their children themselves.

- Children should be informed about what happens to them, helped with decisions that affect them and have their wishes taken into account.

- Children should be safe and protected by effective intervention if they are in danger.

- Court orders should be made only as a last resort.

- Parents continue to have parental responsibility for their children even when they are no longer living with them. They should be kept informed about the children and participate when decisions are being made about the children's future.

- Consideration should be given to children's race, religion, culture and language.

**Parental responsibility:**

- If a child's mother and father were married to each other at the time of the child's birth, they each have parental responsibility towards that child.

- If a child's mother and father are not married to each other at the time of birth, then:
  - The mother alone has parental responsibility.
  - The father does not have parental responsibility unless he acquires it by obtaining a parental responsibility agreement.

**The Patient's Charter: Services for Children and Young People (HMSO, 1996)**

This set out the rights and expectations of children, including:

- Children must be involved in discussions and decisions about their own health.

- Emotional and developmental needs must be taken into account.

- The provision of a safe and appropriate environment in which to deliver care.

- Information must be available about services and treatment, including risks and alternatives.

- There must be respect for a child's confidentiality and access to health records.

- There must be respect for a child's dignity, privacy, and religious and cultural beliefs.

- They must have questions answered and be spoken to in a way that is easily understood.

**'Gillick' Competencies**

- Once children are judged to have 'sufficient understanding' they should be able to make decisions on important matters for themselves, unless there is some age-specific legislation, e.g. age of consent to sexual activity.

- Parents have rights only in so far as these enable them to exercise responsibilities to benefit their children and that these parental rights last only until the child is competent.

- There is no age limit for a child to be deemed 'competent'.

- If a competent child **refuses** to give consent it may be obtained from someone with parental responsibility.

- However, a person with parental responsibility **cannot** override the consent of a competent child.

## Welfare of Children and Young People in Hospital (HMSO, 1991)

- This is the result of a lengthy process and series of reports including:
  - *The Welfare of Children in Hospital*. Report of the Platt Committee (HMSO, 1959).
  - *Fit for the Future*. Report of the Court Committee (HMSO, 1976).
  - The Children Act (HMSO, 1989).
  - The Education Act (1981).

- It reflects the special needs of children and families.

- Its principles are:
  - Children are admitted into hospital only if care cannot be provided in their homes.
  - Close parental contact should be maintained including during x-ray examinations
  - Accommodation, facilities and staffing should be appropriate to the needs of children, separate from those of adults and adolescents if possible.
  - Respect of privacy.
  - The right to be treated with tact and understanding.
  - Right to information, consistent with age and understanding.

## The Children's National Service Framework

- This was set up to develop new national standards for children and young people across the National Health Service (NHS) and social services. It will ensure that they are able to access the right services and are encouraged to take an active part in decisions about their care.

- The children's taskforce is one of ten established to turn the NHS Plan (2000) into reality. The major programme of work is to oversee the National Service Framework (NSF).

- NSF themes include:
  - co-ordination around the development of children and family
  - empowerment of children, young people and parents
  - standards to ensure partnerships, co-ordinated services and inclusiveness
  - appropriate care for the developmental stage of the child or young person and promotion of the child's well-being
  - play and education included in standards

- access for children, particularly to A&E services
- quality, training and accountability of health care staff and leadership, teamwork and networks for children's health care
- safety: environment, service, decision-making and medicines
- changes in culture, workforce and service delivery
- care in the correct environment; aim to deliver care in children's own homes and avoid hospital admissions
- equity of access (geographical locations).

■ The NSF will be an important way of responding to key challenges facing children's health and will have implications for radiology departments in the future.

*Implications for imaging departments*

## Child protection

■ All departments, in district general hospitals as well as specialist children's units, will come into contact with non-accidental injury/child abuse.

■ It is important for radiographers to have an understanding of child protection issues and hospital policies.

■ All professionals concerned with children's care should work together on a multidisciplinary basis, with shared mutual understanding of aims, objectives and what is good practice. 'Inter-disciplinary work is an essential process in the task of attempting to protect children from abuse' (HMSO, 1989).

■ Definitions of abuse:
- emotional: severe or persistent ill treatment
- neglect: may be exposure to danger or repeated failure to attend to physical and developmental needs of the child
- physical: definite knowledge or reasonable suspicion that injury was inflicted or knowingly not prevented
- sexual: involvement of developmentally immature children and adolescents in sexual activities.

■ Radiographers need support because:
- health care professionals who carry out 'technical' tasks are often forgotten
- it requires a wide range of interpersonal skills to be responsive to parents who are angry or upset
- there is a need to create a child-friendly environment in a technical setting.

■ Specific training should include:
- knowledge of hospital policies for child protection, consent/restraint, child protection proceedings

- interpersonal skills, which are required for working with children and families
- coping strategies for dealing with stressful situations
- recognition of signs of child abuse.

■ 'Hospital policies should take into account the radiographer's task in relation to abused children, (Hancock *et al.*, 1997).

■ 'Radiographers need to be aware of the clinical and radiological manifestations of abuse, including the radiographic traces of old abuse. There are implications for workplace support, for management and for training' (Hancock *et al.*, 1997).

### Informed consent

■ The nature, purpose and risks of the examination must be explained to the child and/or parents in non-technical language taking into account:
- type and purpose of the examination
- the nature and effect of the examination, in broad terms
- the principal risks, benefits and consequences if the examination is not done.

■ The child must be capable of understanding. If not, the parent (or person with parental responsibility) should give consent.

■ The person carrying out the procedure should give an explanation but consent is usually obtained by the clinician who refers the patient.
- A full explanation is paramount, with signing of the consent form of secondary importance. If a patient has not been given sufficient information there may be a breach of duty of care to the patient. The child should be encouraged and helped to understand the importance of the procedure without being unduly coerced into agreement.
- There are two types of consent: (1) implied, as when a child climbs voluntarily onto the x-ray table, and (2) express, when the child or parent gives specific agreement, which can be oral but more usually is written.
- Radiographers need time and an appropriate place to give explanations.
- Radiographers need support and training to enable them to support the child and family at times of disagreement and to more fully understand children's rights.

### Restraint

■ Consent is also required if a child needs to be mechanically restrained by a radiographer during an x-ray examination.

■ Restraint means restriction by mechanical means of the physical force of the limbs, head or body of a patient in order to immobilize or keep under control. This might be for the protection or safety of the child, for painful or unpleasant procedures, or because the child is uncooperative.

■ There are many forms of restraint in radiology departments: sandbags, Bucky band, Velcro straps, special immobilizing equipment (Fig. 11.1), wrapping in sheets or physical force by parents or carers. This used to be an uncontested practice.

■ Radiographers must be aware of the legal position with regard to consent, parental responsibility and hospital policies on restraint.

■ Good practice entails accepting practical alternatives such as play, distraction, coping and relaxation techniques, a child-friendly environment, the provision of information and the use of anaesthetic creams for injections. Figure 11.2 shows an alternative seat that is more child friendly with brightly coloured cushions.

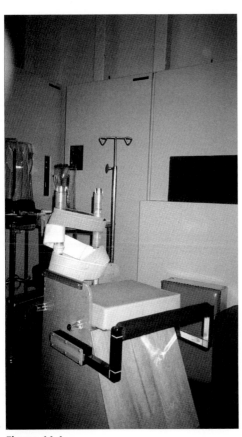

**Figure 11.1**

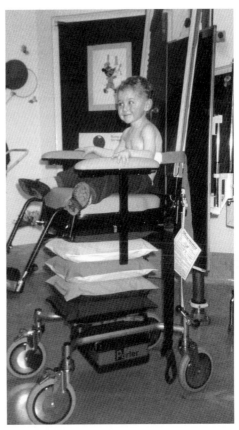

**Figure 11.2**

- A restraint policy for radiography should include:
  - preparation of the child and parents, and the training of staff
  - the child, if competent to understand, should be: (1) advised that restraint is about to take place, (2) given reasons for restraint, and (3) physically prepared to ensure safety, e.g. remove shoes.

- Parents should stay with their child:
  - They should be asked what they would be willing to do to help restrain the child and their idea of acceptable restraining behaviour; it may not be the same for every parent or radiographer.
  - Older children should be asked if they want a parent with them in the x-ray room.

- Restraint must only be used when it is in the best interests of the child.

- Radiographers must know where to obtain further advice and help.

**Other implications for radiology departments**

- The provision of child- and family-centred radiographic services, as already described.

- An environment, facilities and staff that are commensurate with the needs of the child (Fig. 11.3). This should also include privacy and appropriate child-sized gowns (Fig. 11.4).

- The provision of information (Fig. 11.5), incorporating information for children from different ethnic backgrounds.

- Sensitivity to minority groups, such as religious beliefs, feeding and methods of comforting.

- Allowing parents to be with the child at all times.

- A forum for collecting complaints from children.

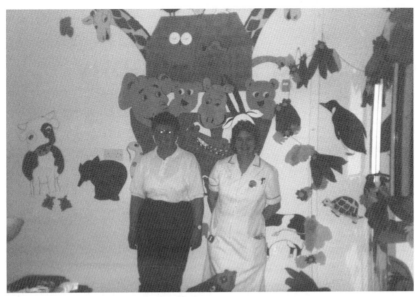

**Figure 11.3**

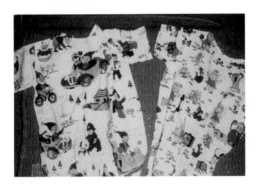

**Figure 11.4**

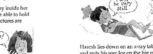

**Figure 11.5**

# References and Bibliography

Association for the Care of Childrens' Health (1992) *Caring for Families and Children.*

British Society of Paediatric Radiology (2003) Draft Standard for skeletal surveys in suspected non-accidental injury (NAI) in children (http://www.bspr.org.uk.nai.htm).

Carty H, Brunelle F, Shaw D, Kendall B (1994) *Imaging Children.* Edinburgh: Churchill Livingstone.

DeLacey G, Guilding A, Wignall B, Reidy J, Bradbrook S (1980) Mild head injuries – a source of excessive radiography? *Clin Radiol* **31**: 457–62.

Gyll C (1983) Design for a paediatric chest stand. *Radiography* **49**(588): 291–3.

Gyll C, Blake N (1986) *Paediatric Diagnostic Imaging.* London: Heinemann Medical Books.

Hadfield JA (1978) *Childhood and Adolescence.* Harmondsworth, UK: Penguin.

HMSO (1959) *Welfare of Children in Hospital Report of the Platt Committee.* London: HMSO, Ministry of Health.

HMSO (1976) *Fit for the Future: Report of the Court Committee on Child Health Services.* London: HMSO, Department of Health and Social Security.

HMSO (1989) *The Children Act.* London: HMSO.

HMSO (1991) *Welfare of Children and Young People in Hospital.* London: HMSO, Department of Health.

HMSO (1996) *The Patient's Charter: Services for Children and Young People.* London: HMSO, Department of Health.

HMSO (2000) *Ionising Radiations (Medical Exposures) Regulations.* London: HMSO, Department of Health.

International Commission for Radiation Protection 14 (1969) Table 1i, Appendix I. *Radiation Cataract in Man.*

Meerstadt PWD, Gyll C (1994) *Manual of Neonatal Emergency Interpretation.* London: WB Saunders.

Raby N, Berman L, De Lacey G (1995) *Accident and Emergency Radiology.* London: WB Saunders.

Rockwood CA, Wilkins KE, King RE (1996) *Fractures in Children*, 4th edn. Philadelphia: Lippincott.

Royal College of Radiologists Working Party (1995) *Making the Best Use of a Department of Clinical Radiology: Guidelines for Doctors*, 3rd edn. London: Royal College of Radiologists.

Save the Children Fund Report (1989) *Hospital: A Deprived Environment for Children.* Save the Children Fund.

Stripp WJ (1979) *Special Techniques in Orthopaedic Radiography.* Edinburgh: Churchill Livingstone.

Thornton A, Gyll C (1999) *Children's Fractures: A Radiological Guide to Safe Practice.* London: WB Saunders.

Tidey B (1995) Metal detector tested as alternative to x-rays. *Radiography* magazine (page 25).

United Nations (1989) *Convention on the Rights of the Child.* Geneva: UN.

Woolf S (1981) *Children under Stress.* Harmondsworth, UK: Penguin.

World Health Organization (1987) *Rational Use of Diagnostic Imaging in Paediatrics.* Technical Report Series 757. Geneva: WHO.

# Index